Treatment Options in Early Intervention

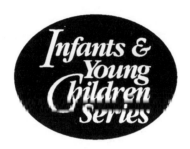

Infants & Young Children Series

Edited by

James A. Blackman, MD, MPH

Professor of Pediatrics
Director of Research
Kluge Children's Rehabilitation Center and Research Institute
Department of Pediatrics
University of Virginia
Charlottesville, Virginia

AN ASPEN PUBLICATION®
Aspen Publishers, Inc.
Gaithersburg, Maryland
1995

Library of Congress Cataloging-in-Publication Data

Treatment options in early intervention / edited by James A. Blackman.
p.   cm.
Articles reprinted from infants and young children.
Includes bibliographical references and index.
ISBN 0-8342-0645-5
1. Handicapped children—Rehabilitation. 2. Child development
deviations—Treatment. I. Blackman, James A.
Infants and young children. II. Infants and young children.
[DNLM: 1. Child Development Disorders—prevention & control—collected works.
2. Child Behavior Disorders—prevention & control—collected works.
WS 350.6 T7847 1995]
RJ138.T74   1995
618.92—dc20
DNLM/DLC
for Library of Congress
94-38449
CIP

Editorial Resources: Amy Myers-Payne

Library of Congress Catalog Card Number: 94-38449
ISBN: 0-8342-0645-5
Series ISBN: 0-8342-0652-8

Printed in the United States of America

1   2   3   4   5

Table of Contents

Preface

Martha is six months old. She was born at 26 weeks gestation, had a moderately stormy newborn intensive care unit experience, and now resides with her 17-year-old single mother who is in a drug rehabilitation program. While Martha is somewhat hypotonic, no definitive developmental diagnosis has been made. Nevertheless, she is considered to be developmentally at-risk because of multiple risk factors. What array of early intervention services, if any, should be offered to this child and her mother?

Traditionally, early intervention was education-focused with emphasis on the child. The common model was for an early childhood educator to visit a home and play with an infant or toddler, often using materials from assessment instruments, in hopes of stimulating the acquisition of new developmental skills.

It became obvious one hour per week had limited impact unless the parent was integrally involved in the visit. Rather than teaching the child, the more sensible goal was to model developmentally appropriate interaction with the child, adapted to meet the child's—and the parent's—unique needs. If a toddler is unable to meet the environment, that is reach for a toy or investigate a cupboard full of pots and pans, because of motor impairment, parents learn how to bring the environment to the child. If an infant is cranky because of an overly sensitive nervous system from asphyxia at birth, the early interventionist demonstrates how to soothe through swaddling, special positioning and handling, and use of a pacifier. If a mother is preoccupied with an unstable, perhaps abusive, relationship with her companion, assistance is provided to seek counseling and protection so that more attention can be given to her child.

From this viewpoint, the dimensions of early intervention expand exponentially. Although attainment of full developmental potential is our mission, strictly developmental interventions form only a part of our task. Health, housing, income, security, and transportation are other necessities without which developmental interventions will be less successful.

Fortunately, Public Law 99-457 (IDEA) promotes early intervention in these broad terms, identifies a wide array of professionals who may need to be involved, and calls for coordination of these services so that families are not overwhelmed by complexity and more red tape. How this can be done is not spelled out in the legislation. How do we overcome years of disciplinary isolation and categorical programming?

The volume provides ideas about specific interventions as well as more general comprehensive intervention strategies. Because most states are on a fast track to full implementation of early intervention services, we cannot afford to duplicate efforts. Learning from others' successes—and failures—will move the process along and bring the benefits of collective wisdom to the front line as quickly as possible.

James A. Blackman, MD, MPH
Editor

Neurodevelopmental treatment (NDT): Therapeutic intervention and its efficacy

Francine Martin Stern, BS, PT
Consultant
Department of Rehabilitation
    Medicine

Delia Gorga, PhD, OTR
Assistant Professor of Rehabilitation
    Medicine
Cornell University Medical College
The New York Hospital-Cornell
    Medical Center
New York, New York

SOME 40 YEARS ago, Karel Bobath, MD and his wife, Berta, a physiotherapist, began questioning the standard treatment of movement disorders for neurologically impaired adults and children. Their ongoing investigations and subsequent treatment philosophy have evolved into what is known throughout the world as the Bobath Method, and in North America, as neurodevelopmental treatment (NDT).[1-6]

What particularly interested Mrs. Bobath was the question, "How can I teach someone to move?" It did not seem reasonable to her that a person with abnormal reflexes and spastic muscles could imitate what a normal body could do.[1] How, for example, could a floppy child understand a command like "put your right leg out," or "straighten your elbow" when he or she never experienced a straight elbow and has no memory of what that feeling is like? By the same token, if someone with poor posture is told to stand up straight, he or she will do so, but only while being observed. A person with good posture, on the other hand, does not have to think about it. In other words, Mrs. Bobath observed, we do not think to move; we do it automatically.

Mrs. Bobath recognized that the spastic child suffers from a "poverty of movement patterns," and that his or her stereotyped movements rely on pathological reflex initiation, which eventually leads to deformity. The child's muscles may only appear to be weak because they cannot function optimally due to the spasticity or tightness of the opposing muscle.[1-6] Also, the more the child tries, the more spastic he or she gets and eventually he or she may give up in frustration.

RELATIONSHIP OF MOVEMENT AND LEARNING

So, philosophically, the NDT approach began to differ considerably from the orthopedic-rehabilitation concept that stresses compensating for what one cannot use (the affected parts) by what one can, for example, teaching a spastic child with long leg braces to walk by using his or her arms and leaning on crutches. From an NDT perspective, it became clear that the chief difficulty for the handicapped child was to receive and integrate environmental information and then to coordi-

The project on which this article is based was funded by the Pain Control Fund of the Department of Rehabilitation Medicine at The New York Hospital-Cornell Medical Center.

Inf Young Children 1988; 1(1): 22–32

1

nate the responses to allow him or her to interact with the environment. Secondly, it was important to take into consideration the vital relationship between movement and learning.[3–7]

Every combination of movement is practiced by an infant.[2] At first, the new activity may be clumsy but through a process of trial and error the infant will modify and adapt his or her sensory-motor experiences and learn the new activity. But in order to get movement, balance and posture in space must be flexible, and in order for that to happen an infant needs enough tone or stability to make weight bearing against gravity possible. For example, the postural tone cannot be so high (spastic) as to interfere with movement or too low (floppy) or unsteady (athetoid) so as to be unable to support a movement.[4] Imagine standing in a moving subway car. You cannot rigidly lock your knees or you will fall, but you have to be flexible enough to quickly adjust when the train lurches. Children with these problems get "stuck" using abnormal patterns to move or to stabilize, which prohibit further movement. The aim of NDT is to give a person all possible mobility during treatment and help him or her develop, without excessive effort, control over his or her abnormal patterns in order to obtain more function.

NDT AND NEUROLOGICAL AND DEVELOPMENTAL DEFICITS

This new way of looking at movement disorders is called NDT because of the two main deficits that have to be taken into account when studying children: the neurological and the developmental.[1–6] A lesion in the brain produces abnormal reflex activity resulting in abnormal postures and patterns as well as a delay in the maturation of the brain. Therefore, it is important to coordinate stopping, or "inhibiting" the abnormal with the process of allowing normal movement to occur, or "facilitating."[8] From a foundation of more normal tone, gained by using techniques of inhibition and facilitation, the therapist can elicit righting and equilibrium reactions, which are the foundation of normal posture and movement.[5]

There are many different ways of inhibiting abnormal muscle tone and facilitating normal movement reactions, depending on the type of pattern and distribution of pathology. A child may be floppy in his or her trunk with spasticity in his or her limbs, or be rigid, and then quickly change to alternating tone. The therapist must have an understanding of normal and abnormal movement in order to know what technique will be successful and when to use it.

GOALS OF NDT

The goals of NDT can be listed as follows:[9]
- To carefully analyze problems of posture and movement in all possible positions;

- To normalize tone using techniques of inhibition and facilitation in order to allow the child to move more functionally;
- To teach parents and teachers the necessary procedures to ensure consistent management of motor deficits;
- To use equipment to aid in enabling more normal patterns of movement and to help in functional skills; and
- To prevent a cycle of abnormal sensory motor development including secondary changes such as contractures and deformities from occurring.

All of these goals sound complicated and are often difficult to explain in a brief summary, but perhaps some graphic illustrations will help. Fig 1a is a picture of a 6-month-old infant. He is unable to lift his head correctly against gravity, his arms are retracted, and he cannot position his elbows under his shoulders. Fig 1b shows the same infant lying on a soft roll. His arms are elongated and now he is able to lift his head (righting reaction) in response to the environmental input. This may

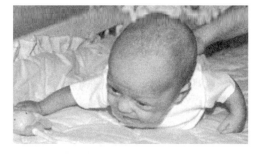

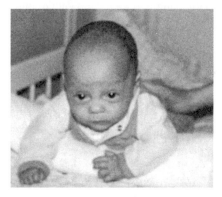

Fig 1. (a) Six-month-old infant, unable to lift his head against gravity, with retracted arms, and unable to position his elbows under his shoulders. **(b)** The same infant, lying on a soft roll. His arms are elongated and he is able to lift his head in response to environmental input.

be called positioning, but it is also active therapy because the child is responding by himself in a correct functional pattern that he can practice on his own.

Fig 2a is a 1-year-old with spastic diplegia who sits unsupported on the floor. Her spine is rounded and abnormal tone causes excessive backward tipping of the pelvis and abnormal extension patterns of the lower extremities. Fig 2b is the same child in unsupported sitting after one session of NDT.

Fig 3a is a child standing alone, before therapy. Her legs are pulled into patterns of scissoring and internal rotation at the hip. In Figs 3b and 3c, following therapy, she can come up to stand with minimal facilitation using a normal reciprocal disassociated pattern, that is to say, she separates her legs and stands up on one at a time.

Fig 4a is a 6-month-old spastic quadriplegic infant lying on his back. Due to excessive extensor tone and abnormal reflexes he cannot keep his head midline or reach forward to grasp a toy. Fig 4b shows his mother practicing handling techniques that enable her child to move successfully and interact with her. He can now reach midline and grab his feet.

The central nervous system is influenced by treating the child's reaction to handling. Infants best communicate motorically; their motor systems are a clue to their behavior, a window to their neurological functioning.[10] Therefore, we all need to become better observors. Being intimately familiar with the patterns of pathology seen in older children with cerebral palsy makes it easier to spot the subtler deviations demonstrated by younger children.

THE EVALUATION PROCESS

When one is evaluating an infant or a young child, one is evaluating a process that is a dynamic interaction. "If I move you this way, how will you respond? Are you frightened? Do you have to clench your hands? Why do you fall into gravity? Are you stiff? Can you see the toy?" and most important of all, "Can you change?" Age may not make as much of a difference as changeability, which is the most important factor in making a good prognosis for the future.[11] If practitioners can prevent a child from getting "stuck" that much longer, it will be possible to keep him or her free to learn. In other words, during treatment (and assessment) practitioners communicate the possibilities of movement to the child so that he or she feels and learns it in the most natural way. Immediate improvement of tone and active movement in any one treatment session should be possible, and only those techniques that work should continue to be used. The developmental sequence is of secondary importance and may not necessarily be followed. There are often advantages to skipping a step (crawling, for example) and coming back to it later. Very few infants actually perfect a milestone before they move on to another.[7,8,12,13]

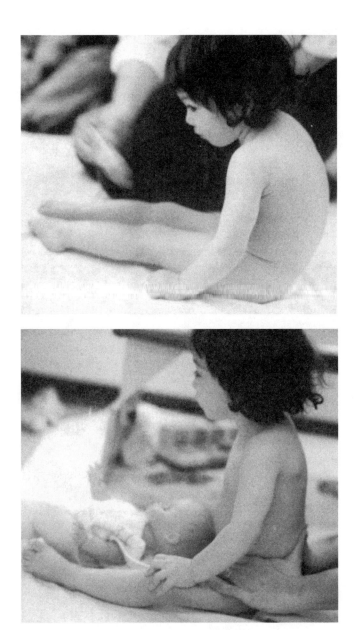

Fig 2. (a) One-year-old with spastic diplegia. Her spine is rounded and abnormal tone causes backward tipping of the pelvis and abnormal extension patterns of the lower extremities. **(b)** Same child in unsupported sitting after one session of NDT.

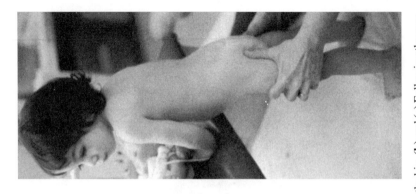

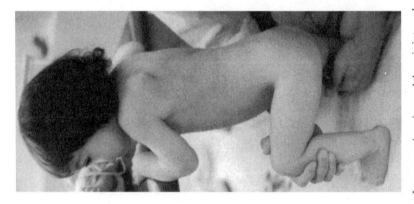

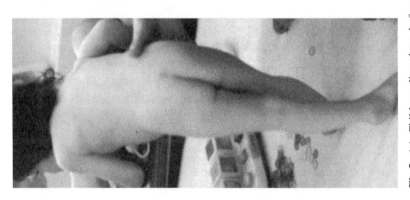

Fig 3. (a) Child standing alone, before therapy. Legs are scissoring and there is internal rotation at the hip. (b) and (c) Following therapy, child can stand with minimal facilitation using a normal reciprocal disassociated pattern.

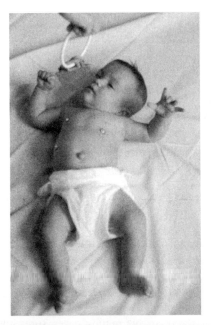

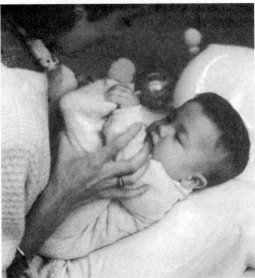

Fig 4. (a) Six-month-old spastic quadriplegic infant lying on his back. Due to excessive extensor tone and abnormal reflexes he cannot keep his head midline or reach forward to grasp a toy. **(b)** Same infant with his mother, practicing handling techniques that enable the child to reach midline and grab his feet.

As in any good treatment approach, a thorough assessment of the child must be made. In order to determine what is preventing normal tone and movement and to plan how they should be treated, assessment should be ongoing, adjusted to the needs of each individual child, and changed along with the child. Although cerebral palsy is caused by a static, nonprogressive lesion of the brain, the clinical manifestations of this disorder are not static and vary considerably within the same child and among children. Tone changes with position, direction against gravity, even with moods such as excitement or fatigue. The cerebral palsy child has a narrower range of possibilities and less control over these fluctuations so that increasing the range and grading of a movement becomes that much more significant.

As treatment progresses, less and less guidance by the therapist is necessary and the child begins to take over. Treatment goals must be set that are realistic, reachable, and that lead easily to the next higher goal. There are no lists of exercises or drills to practice. The therapist becomes the monitor of postural control (dynamic biofeedback), finding the child's potential by his or her reaction to movement and teaching him or her to automatically control it.[7] Thus, the whole child is treated, not one muscle in isolation. The child learns normal movement in a context of functional activity. The end result of therapy, of course, will be determined by the extent of the damage to the brain, but in most cases, some intervention should be continued through the growing years.

ROLE OF EACH THERAPY DISCIPLINE

Each therapy discipline, physical therapy, occupational therapy, and speech therapy has its own expertise in NDT, but the boundaries are very flexible. Traditionally the physical therapist concentrates on gross motor activities, the occupational therapist on fine motor and play, and the speech therapist on feeding skills and prespeech. But, because of the nature of the handicap in cerebral palsy, all three therapists need to create a background of normal tone for each child in order to build the child's skills. Therefore, the therapists may actually use the same techniques to prepare the child in order to achieve the goals of their specific discipline. When more than one discipline is working with the child, communication among the therapists is essential.

One of the primary goals of NDT is to provide a consistent carry over into all of a child's daily activities and to increase his or her range of normal sensory experience. Children learn through their senses, and the mother, or primary caretaker, has a lot of opportunity for purposeful therapeutic handling during dressing, feeding, and play.[9] The importance of instructing parents in home management skills and the necessity for sensitizing them in how to recognize and differentiate between normal and abnormal patterns of movement cannot be overemphasized.

Special handling skills must come spontaneously and naturally from parents just as other elements of their repertoire of good parenting, and not as therapeutic regimens. For this reason, we emphasize teaching these skills early on, with the goal of ensuring that they become a part of the parents' automatic physical interaction with the child. By the same token, all teachers and therapists who come in contact with the child should be reliable and consistent in their approach in order to ensure a satisfactory emotional and social adjustment.

NDT IS APPLICABLE TO MANY DISABILITIES

At this point, it is important to mention that NDT is a movement-learning approach that can be applied to persons with all types of disabilities. The emphasis on detailed movement assessment and the importance of treatment of the whole body and not just one limb or muscle in isolation, makes NDT an ideal treatment approach for many orthopedic and neuromuscular patients. A postfracture patient, for example, just out of a long-leg cast, can be treated sitting on a ball to feel weight shift on the injured leg, can practice automatic balance reactions, and can respond with associated unused muscles. In this case, the NDT approach would enhance the rehabilitation process by providing a thorough and functional therapeutic program.

NDT training courses range from the basic eight-week certification course or a three-week adult hemiplegia certification course, to advanced courses in such subjects as prespeech and feeding, baby, and upper-extremity function. According to the Neuro-Developmental Treatment Association of Oak Park, Illinois, the courses are open to therapists—physical, occupational, and speech—as well as to teachers and physicians. Pediatricians and pediatric neurologists should be aware of the types of intervention programs available to their patients and the type of training of the personnel. There are many differences in programs and differences between one center and another. Each one will reflect its own treatment philosophy and emphasis.[14] The suitability of any one treatment for a particular child depends on many factors—the type of problem or age of the patient, for example. One center may offer group therapy sessions where a therapist is a guide and demonstrates handling techniques to the caretakers, while another center may provide one-on-one hourly therapy sessions.

THE EFFICACY OF NDT

There is no conclusive evidence that NDT works, but on the other hand there is no conclusive evidence that NDT does not work. This is a simplistic view of a very complex problem. Despite absence of conclusive evidence based on rigorous research studying the effectiveness of NDT,[15-22] there is a consensus among parents

and therapists experienced with the approach that the treatment makes a difference. If one were to ask a group of parents whose children received therapy
whether they felt that therapy helped their children, they may react in different
ways: their child "loosened up," became more mobile and independent, less fearful of movement, gained better balance, became more erect. When parents consider changes in themselves, they might remark that they felt more positive toward
their child, felt more involved in their child's development, understood their
child's needs, felt it helped them focus on the "here and now," and felt they were
not alone with their problem. If one were to ask therapists treating motorically
handicapped children if therapy makes a difference, similar responses would be
made.

Why then is it so difficult to document the positive effect of NDT from research
studies when a consensus among parents and therapists involved in the process
persists? The problems are many and range from those inherent in designing behavioral research[23] and the actual focus of the studies.

One of the problems in interpreting the results of intervention studies is that it
has not been feasible to determine which variable was responsible for a change in
the child's motor function: therapy, the environment, neurological maturation, or
the nature of the child's brain lesion. It is difficult to hold any of these variables
constant so that cause and effect can be established. No two children have exactly
the same environment, rate of neurological maturation, or brain lesion. Even the
type of treatment differs from therapist to therapist based on their own experience
and skill. It is particularly difficult, then, to dispel the notion that the child may
have outgrown the problem rather than attribute the improvement to treatment
intervention.

Another problem in documenting treatment effectiveness is the method used to
identify motor change in each child. The tools are often quantitative indicators of
motor development based on the acquisition of motor milestones. Tests such as
the Bayley Infant Scales measure the presence or absence of age-appropriate motor abilities such as sitting independently.[24] The test does not account for the quality of the movement, that is, how the infant accomplishes a task. For example, the
child may pass the item, "sits independently," but does so with a rounded back and
stiff legs. In the NDT approach, measuring the quality of movement is a significant objective. To date, few studies have addressed this aspect of treatment
change.[25]

For some children in therapy, the capacity for achieving normal motor milestones may be limited and the rate at which they reach the milestones unpredictable. However, a change may be seen in the quality of movement in response to
therapy. For example, if a treatment study were undertaken over a 12-month period, a child may not achieve independent sitting by the end of that time period;
however, he or she may develop better trunk extension, improved balance in sit-

ting, freer use of his or her upper extremities in the supported sitting position, or increased pelvic mobility. All these aspects contribute to the quality of a child's sitting, yet are not measured using conventional motor development testing methods. Changes in motor status may also occur in smaller increments that current testing methods may be insensitive to.

Perhaps the emphasis on the acquisition of motor milestones, rather than on the improvement of movement quality stems from the conventional way in which some professionals define a positive outcome or goal. For example, a physician may ask, "Is Peter walking yet?" The NDT therapist may reply, that although Peter may not be walking independently and still has cerebral palsy, he is symmetrical, is beginning to develop balance in standing, and uses less compensatory movements of his trunk when walking. While these quality changes may affect the child's function, progress is only viewed by how soon the child has achieved the next step toward motor independence, rather than achievement of the intermediary steps. Often, unrealistic goals are set that then may negate the positive influence of therapy. A child may never walk without support, but that does not necessarily mean that the therapy was not effective.

One might ask then, why alternative methods are not used in the research design instead of testing with less sensitive measures. Assessment methods used by clinicians are usually descriptive and have not been subjected to the rigors of psychometric test construction. As a result, at this point, they could not be used for research until they were well-validated, demonstrated as reliable, and possibly standardized. Although many clinicians and researchers in the therapy fields are presently working on test development,[26–29] few are ready to be used in research studies.

Treatment studies may also be considered narrow in their focus if the objective of the studies is only determining the extent of change in the child's motor function. There are many other aspects of treatment that contribute to the ultimate outcome of the child's physical abilities and are usually not included in the studies to date. For example, a vital part of treatment is how the child is handled at home and in school. It is not only his or her individual treatment with the therapist that will influence development, but how parents and caregivers incorporate the objectives of the treatment into daily care. While this information on how effective parents have become in influencing motor patterns through their handling is part of every clinical assessment, this information is not usually gathered in research studies. By including measurement of changes in handling, interpretation of research results would be enhanced by beginning to explain the influence of the environment, specifically parent handling, on motor progress.

Finally, the influence of the NDT approach on parent attitude and parent–child interaction should not be underestimated. While one might argue that other treatment approaches would include providing parent support and guidance through the process, helping parents understand their child's needs and demonstrating the methods to change their handling and the child's environment are part of the cornerstone of the NDT philosophy of treatment. The gains in parents' emotional growth that may have a pervasive effect on their child's progress have not been tapped in current research studies.

•   •   •

NDT treatment is constantly changing, not only to suit the need of the individual patient, but on a larger scale, as it adapts and integrates into the skills of individual therapists, teachers, parents, and physicians. There is a tremendous need for better interdisciplinary research to increase the understanding of child development, detection, and intervention of disabled children.

REFERENCES

1. Bobath K: *Abnormal Postural Reflex Activity Caused by Brain Lesions.* London, W.S. Heinemann, 1964.
2. Bobath B: The very early treatment of cerebral palsy. *Dev Med Child Neur* 1967;9:373–390.
3. Bobath B: Motor development, its effect on general development, and application to the treatment of cerebral palsy. *Physiotherapy* 1971;57:526–532.
4. Bobath B: *Motor Development in the Different Types of Cerebral Palsy.* London, W.S. Heinemann, 1975.
5. Bobath B: *Adult Hemiplegia. Evaluation and Treatment.* London, W.S. Heinemann, 1978.
6. Bobath K: *A Neurophysiological Basis for the Treatment of Cerebral Palsy.* London, W.S. Heinemann, 1980.
7. Scherzer A, Tscharnuter, I: *Early Diagnosis and Therapy in Cerebral Palsy.* New York, Marcel Dekker, 1982.
8. Bryce D: Facilitation of movement—Bobath approach. *Physiotherapy* 1972;58:403–407.
9. Campbell P: *Introduction to Neurodevelopmental Treatment.* Akron, Ohio, Childrens Hospital Medical Center of Akron and Kent State University. Monograph, 1986.
10. Wolf P: The relationship of neuromotor maturation on psychological development. Paper presentation, *Issues in Infant Development*, Contemporary Forums Conference, New York, NY, May 11–13, 1987.
11. Stern FM: Screening the high risk infant in a follow-up program. *Totline* 1987;13:24–25.
12. Corner FP, Williamson GG, Siepp JM (eds): *Program Guide for Infants and Toddlers with Neuromotor and other Developmental Disabilities.* New York, Teachers College Press, 1978.
13. Finnie NR: *Handling the Cerebral Palsy Child At Home.* London, W.S. Heinemann, 1974.
14. Scrutten D (ed): *Management of the Motor Disorders of Children with Cerebral Palsy.* London, Spastics International Medical Publications, 1984.
15. Carlson PN: Comparison of two occupational therapy approaches for teaching the young cerebral-palsied child. *Am J Occup Ther* 1975;29:267–272.
16. Goodman M, Rothberg AD, Houston-McMillan JE, et al: Effects of early neurodevelopmental

therapy in normal and at-risk survivors of neonatal intensive care. *Lancet* 1985;2:1327–1330.

17. Harris SR: Effects of neurodevelopmental therapy on motor performance of infants with Down's Syndrome. *Dev Med Child Neur* 1981;23:477–483.

18. Hourcade J, Parette P: Motoric changes subsequent to therapeutic intervention in infants and young children who have cerebral palsy: An annotated listing of group studies. *Percept Mot Skills* 1984;58(2):519–524.

19. Kong E: Very early treatment of cerebral palsy. *Dev Med Child Neur* 1966;8:198–222.

20. Ottenbacher KJ, Biocca Z, De Cremer G, et al: Quantitative analysis of the effectiveness of pediatric therapy. Emphasis on the Neurodevelopmental Approach. *Phy Ther* 1986;66:1095–1101.

21. Piper MC, Mazer BC, Hardy S, et al: Monitoring the effects of early physical therapy on the high risk infant: A preliminary report. *Phys Occup Ther Pediatr* 1986;6:303–318.

22. Piper MC, Kunos VI, Willis DM, et al: Early physical therapy effects on the high-risk infant. A randomized controlled trial. *Pediatrics* 1986;78:216–224.

23. Kerlinger FN: *Foundations of Behavioral Research.* New York, Holt, Rinehart & Winston, 1965.

24. Bayley N: *Bayley Scales of Infant Development.* New York, Psychological Corporation, 1969.

25. DeGangi GA, Hurley L, Linscheid TR: Toward a methodology of the short-term effects of neurodevelopmental treatment. *Am J Occup Ther* 1983;37:479–484.

26. Georgo H, Stern HM, Ross CF: Trends in neuromotor behavior of preterm and full term infants in the first year of life: A preliminary report. *Dev Med Child Neur* 1985;2/!:156–166.

27. Harris SR: Early detection of CP: Sensitivity and specificity of 2 motor assessment tools. *J Perinatol* 1987;7(1):11–15.

28. Harris SR, Brady DK: Infant neuromotor assessment instruments: A review. *Phys Occup Ther Pediatr* 1986;6:121–153.

29. Harris SM, Heriza CB: Measuring infant movement. *Phys Ther* 1987;67:1877–1880.

Tracheostomy in young children: Implications for assessment and treatment of communication and feeding disorders

Bonnie M. Simon, MA, CCC-SP
Speech–Language Pathologist
United Cerebral Palsy Association
Northwest Center Home Health
  Agency
Private Practice
Huntingdon Valley, Pennsylvania

**Joy Silverman McGowan, MS,
  CCC-SP**
Speech–Language Pathologist
Division of Communication Disorders
Children's Seashore House
Philadelphia, Pennsylvania

WITHIN THE PAST decade improvements in medical technology have resulted in the presence of a unique population of infants surviving severe medical complications. This group of infants and young children include those requiring placement of the tracheostomy. Previous management by physicians has focused primarily on medical concerns without consideration for the effect of tracheostomy on the child's overall communication and feeding development. If the tracheostomy placement is of short duration (3 to 4 weeks) and if the child is able to vocalize around the tracheostomy tube, then developmental communicative issues may be less critical. However, associated feeding difficulties resulting from the tracheostomy placement warrant immediate intervention.

Recent studies have concluded that children with long-term tracheostomies may be at risk for developmental delay that may include communicative and feeding impairments.[1-5] The children with long-term tracheostomies, for as long as one month to several years, are likely to need continual intervention throughout the period of cannulation.

Since the primary physician may have more frequent and direct contact with the infants and their families, it is important to recognize the child's developmental needs and to provide appropriate guidance in facilitating early intervention for communication and feeding issues.[6] It is hoped that this article will provide information to assist all professionals in the management of communication and feeding disorders for tracheostomized children in an effort to decrease the frustration felt by the family or caregiver as well as that felt by the children.

MEDICAL CONSIDERATIONS

The presence of the tracheostomy tube allows for pulmonary toilet, mechanical ventilation, and the bypass of an upper-airway obstruction. The conditions requiring placement of the tracheostomy in infants are the following:

Inf Young Children 1989; 1(3):1–9
© 1989 Aspen Publishers, Inc.

- ventilator dependence;
- subglottic stenosis (narrowing of the airway beneath the glottis);
- tracheomalacia (softening of the cartilage of the trachea);
- tracheoesophageal anomalies;
- neuromuscular disorders;
- congenital anomalies;
- craniofacial anomalies;
- laryngeal neoplasm (laryngeal growth or tumor);
- cardiac anomalies;
- croup; and
- epiglottitis (inflammation of the epiglottis).

The actual placement of the tracheostomy is through an incision within the third tracheal ring. A tracheostomy tube, or cannula, is inserted into the trachea to allow a patent airway. Although many infants may require short-term tracheostomy placement, it is often found that premature infants with a diagnosis of bronchopulmonary dysplasia may develop a condition of subglottic stenosis requiring long-term cannulation with or without ventilator dependence.

In addition, many infants may require tracheostomy placement as a result of structural abnormalities, such as tracheomalacia, tracheoesophageal anomalies, or laryngeal neoplasm. Those children experiencing congenital or craniofacial anomalies may require placement of a tracheostomy until maturational growth changes occur or until surgical procedures are performed to improve the patency of the airway, allowing normal respiratory functioning. Infants with cardiac anomalies, croup, and epiglottitis may require variable periods of cannulation, depending on the severity and nature of their illness.

Children with the additional problem of a neuromuscular disorder can require lengthier periods of cannulation, depending on the extent of their neurologic involvement. For example, children with a diagnosis of myopathy or severe neuromuscular disorders may require permanent tracheostomy placement with a more intensive habilitative program.

EARLY COMMUNICATION NEEDS

The development of speech and language in the tracheostomized child has been found to be related to the time of cannulation.[6] If the child receives a tracheostomy during the prelinguistic stage of development (prior to the development of meaningful language), then speech and language therapy may be needed for both the establishment of a communication system and for early vocal production.

The quality of parent–child interaction is affected when an infant is unable to engage in turn-taking vocal play in response to the parent's attention. When a child experiences a prolonged period of aphonia, it is crucial to facilitate parent–

child interaction by training the parent to encourage and to reinforce nonverbal, gestural cues and attending behaviors.

VOICE PRODUCTION

Speech and language therapy may be needed for both the development of a communication system and for establishing early vocal productions. To produce a voice, a leak of air must pass around the cannula to the level of the vocal cords (Fig 1). Once the cannula is placed within the trachea, the size and fit of the cannula may prohibit air from passing up to the level of the vocal cords, resulting in absent or inconsistent vocalizations. If the cannula fits tightly within the tracheal airway, then the air leak is usually absent (Fig 2). Thus the condition of aphonia (absence of voice) occurs. Children with neuromuscular difficulties or mild hypotonia may also exhibit a period of aphonia, even if an air leak is present within the laryngeal airway. These neurologically impaired children may require intensive speech therapy in an effort to obtain respiratory–phonatory coordination.

For young tracheostomized children, specific techniques may be used to stimulate babbling experiences. Some children learn spontaneous use of tongue clicks or buccal speech,[6] but these methods are not felt to be an effective communication system.

Occlusion of the cannula may be taught to initiate vocalizations. Intermittent attempts of occlusion, for a brief period of time (1 to 3 seconds), may result in the emittance of vocalizations. If infants are provided with auditory–vocal feedback,

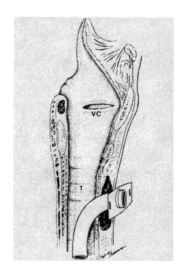

Fig 1. Tracheostomy cannula in place in cervical trachea. Reprinted with permission from Simon BM, Handler SD: The speech pathologist and management of children with tracheostomies. *J Otolaryngol* 1981;10:441. Copyright (1981, International Journal of Pediatric Oto-Rhino-Laryngology).

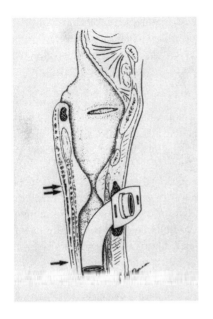

Fig 2. Tight-fitting tracheostomy cannula or subglottic stenosis impeding flow of air across the vocal cords and preventing vocalization. Reprinted with permission from Simon BM, Handler SD: The speech pathologist and management of children with tracheostomies. *J Otolaryngol* 1981;10:442. Copyright (1981, International Journal of Pediatric Oto-Rhino-Laryngology).

the possibility of more frequent vocal attempts may occur. Some young children may learn independent occlusion of the cannula to produce vocalizations by 1 to 2 years of age. Initially clinicians may feel uncomfortable occluding the cannula. As an alternative to the direct occlusion, clinicians can model the occlusion on their own neck while reinforcing the child's independent occlusion when imitated. When occluding the cannula careful monitoring by a physician, a trained family member, or a nurse is suggested to avoid compromising the respiratory status of the child.

Clinicians and parents should be cautioned in attempting to occlude the cannula. When the cannula is tight fitting, this occlusion, coupled with a forced, effortful, vocal attempt, may result in the condition of subcutaneous emphysema (the presence of air in the subcutaneous tissue).

It is possible for infants to develop spontaneous vocalizations without providing occlusion of the cannula during various periods of the cannulation. Intermittent or inconsistent vocalizations may result from alterations in cannula size, structural changes in the airway, or changes in ventilator settings. Infants and children requiring mechanical ventilation have often been more successful in obtaining vocalizations. If children require a high inspiratory pressure to inflate their lungs, this increased pressure can aid in the emergence of vocalizations with the presence of an air leak around the tracheostomy tube. It is important to be aware that vocalizations emitted with supplemental ventilation are produced on inspiration rather than expiration, as is required for normal phonation. This can be confusing for children who are gradually weaned from the ventilator, requiring constant adjustments of their respiratory mechanisms while learning to produce normal vocalizations.

The fenestrated cannula (Fig 3) has been successful for obtaining vocalizations in some adults with tracheostomies. The fenestrated tube has not been effective for use in infants, since its use of a plastic material deteriorates more readily, causing weakening of the tracheal wall. This may also place the child at risk for the development of tracheal granulomas.

The use of a Passy-Muir tracheostomy speaking valve has been beneficial in promoting normal vocalizations for nonventilator-dependent tracheostomized infants who do not exhibit severe subglottic stenosis or who do not require frequent suctioning.[7] Additionally, the Passy-Muir valve eliminates the need for digital occlusion of the cannula. Although some young children have found this specific valve to be difficult or uncomfortable, others have become desensitized to its use and have initiated more frequent verbal productions.

The Hollinger tracheostomy cannula provides an additional inner cannula that is helpful in obtaining vocalizations. In the authors' experience, however, placement of the inner cannula can cause discomfort to very young children and may impede their vocal attempts. However, experienced clinicians familiar with other types of cannulas, such as the Franklin and the Shiley,[8] may have similar success in obtaining and maintaining vocalizations even without altering the cannula during vocal attempts.

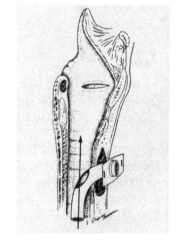

Fig 3. Fenestrated tracheostomy cannula permitting flow of air through cannula and across vocal cords allowing vocalization. Reprinted with permission from Simon BM, Handler SD: The speech pathologist and management of children with tracheostomies. *J Otolaryngol* 1981;10:442. Copyright (1981, International Journal of Pediatric Oto-Rhino-Laryngology).

AUGMENTATIVE/ALTERNATIVE COMMUNICATION

Children who are unable to produce consistent vocalizations for obtaining verbal communication should be considered for an augmentative or alternative communication system. These children are capable of establishing a symbolic system (associating meaning with concepts of objects) at a developmental age level of 9 to 15 months. An augmentative communication system is used to supplement the infant's verbal attempts. An alternative communication system is usually implemented with children who are unable to vocalize. Four forms of augmentative/alternative communication may be suggested for tracheostomized children depending on the specific needs of the child:

1. Signed English
2. Artificial speech through use of an electrolarynx
3. Esophageal speech
4. Manual or electronic communication systems

During the period in which expressive communication is beginning to emerge, sign language may be initiated as an augmentative communication system. Sign language (specifically signed English) is a nonvocal system of gestures most often taught to children who are just initiating a communication system. Signed English is taught rather than American sign language because of its correspondence to spoken-word order. Expressive language can be facilitated through signed English once the child demonstrates a meaningful symbol system. Normal children point and gesture to aid their early communicative attempts, thus providing a basis for sign-language training.[10] Parents should feel confident about accepting this early communication system for their children and should understand that it will be supplemented later with a more natural form of verbal communication once the child demonstrates capabilities for producing speech movements to approximate words.

Verbalizations or vocal stimulation should be encouraged, even in the presence of intermittent vocalizations. When aphonia is present, stimulation of articulatory movements through play interactions may be helpful in facilitating spoken communication. Use of the electrolarynx has been found to be a more easily interpreted system than sign language, even with the high-intensity levels and limited pitch variability found with artificial speech. Use of the electrolarynx has been successful in the hospital environment for children requiring long-term or permanent tracheostomies. During therapeutic speech sessions, the electrolarynx may be a useful method to enable the child to approximate normalized speech movements for the later development of oral communication.

Esophageal speech may be chosen as the primary communication system for children with long-term or permanent tracheostomies and for children who may exhibit capabilities for developing functioning oral–motor postures for verbalizations.[11] This method has also been recommended for children who have severe subglottic stenosis or a laryngeal diversion, conditions that prevent air from passing to the vocal folds. When these tracheolaryngeal conditions occur, children may attempt normal respiratory patterns that could lead to the natural emission of pharyngeal or esophageal productions without the benefit of special training. If these esophageal sounds are reinforced appropriately, a viable communication system may emerge as words are elicited. Training for the development of esophageal speech should follow similar guidelines to those established for training older patients learning to use this mode of communication. However, speech and language stimulation techniques commonly modeled through play situations are strongly suggested to avoid frustration.

Use of an augmentative communication system is recommended for long-term tracheostomized or ventilator-dependent children. Manual or electronic communication devices (with synthesized speech) are usually prescribed for children with severe oral–motor dysfunction and poor speech intelligibility. Special positioning considerations for adaptive seating may be necessary to enable children to access or to use a communication system. Coordinated team management must be implemented to determine the optimal communication system and appropriate positioning.[12]

SPEECH AND LANGUAGE DEVELOPMENT POSTDECANNULATION

Various longitudinal studies have documented the effects of vocal deprivation on tracheostomized infants and young children.[10,13] The development of functional speech and language postdecannulation seems to be related to the development level of speech and language skills at the time of decannulation. The child who has developed a symbolic communication system of words (vocal or nonvocal) is considered to be in the linguistic stage of language development. One who has not developed word usage is considered to be in the prelinguistic stage.

Infants who have been deprived of early vocalizations into their linguistic stage of development may demonstrate significant speech and language delays after decannulation, impeding the development of spoken-word production. Speech and language intervention should include methods that will minimize the level of communicative frustration while training newly learned oral–motor postures for speech production. These children who have benefited from speech and language intervention during cannulation may need less intensive speech therapy if adequate neurologic, medical, and developmental status are seen. Augmentative systems should be maintained throughout the period in which functional expressive communication develops. For children who are able to consistently or intermittently vocalize prior to the development of symbolic communication, speech and language skills may normalize postdecannulation; therefore less intensive therapeutic intervention may be suggested.

Periodic communication assessments and voice evaluations should accompany all developmental diagnostic evaluations. Careful monitoring of voice quality is necessary because of the increased risk of vocal pathology associated with tracheostomized children. Specifically, a high incidence of chronic hoarseness, breathiness, and pitch disturbances have been seen in this population.

Developmental delay has been common among the young tracheostomized population.[14–17] Children with long-term tracheostomies may experience lengthy periods of hospitalization, which may contribute to delayed milestones. Infant stimulation programs within the hospital, community, and home are strongly recommended during the period of cannulation. These programs can provide assessment of developmental needs and can help the child to achieve his or her maximum capabilities for learning.

FEEDING DIFFICULTIES

Children with tracheostomies are at risk for developing feeding difficulties. Dysphagia may occur in association with tracheostomy placement and may interfere with medical management. The presence of the tracheostomy causes structural change within the laryngeal airway. Inhibited laryngeal movement and physical discomfort may be seen with the initial placement of the cannula. Increased tracheal secretions may also contribute to the child's physical discomfort, interrupting his or her mealtimes with frequent suctioning.[10–13]

Children with severe neonatal complications who demonstrate decreased muscle tone may exhibit weakened suckling movements and dysphagia.[18] These infants may be identified as the slow feeders, who require specialized techniques and lengthy feeding sessions. The children may need supplemental nasogastric or gastrostomy tube feedings to maintain adequate weight gain.

Dysphagia is also common in children who exhibit neurologic symptoms. Children with neuromotor involvement may exhibit additional problems, including poor tongue and lip control. These children may often require adaptive positioning to maximize oral feeding experiences. In cases of severe neurologic impairment and ventilator dependency, frequent adjustments in positioning may be necessary to avoid compromising the child's respiratory status during oral feedings. Occasional pauses during mealtimes may be necessary to increase the infant's tolerance to complete feedings. Frequent burping is recommended during bottle feeding for infants who develop abdominal distention, commonly seen in ventilator-dependent infants who exhibit poor sucking movements and take in additional air during bottle feedings.

Prior to initiating a full feeding program, use of methylene blue or dye should be introduced with a bolus to screen for aspiration. If aspiration is felt to be present, videofluorography is then recommended. For tracheostomized infants, a fluoroscopic swallowing function study should include an examination of the oral and pharyngeal aspects of swallowing behavior in addition to esophageal components.[19]

The chronically ill, long-term, hospitalized child may present with oral hypersensitivity if early intervention and oral–motor stimulations are not provided. Oral hypersensitivity may be apparent in children who experience frequent suctioning and who receive noxious stimulation around the mouth. The importance of early feeding experiences (both nutritive and non-nutritive) may decrease the possibility of developing resistance to oral feedings or later behavioral feeding difficulties. Bernbaum et al[20] reported that children who were provided with early oral non-nutritive sucking experiences exhibited increased tolerance for nutritive oral feedings and exhibited more rapid weight gain.

Children exhibiting oral hypersensitivity and prolonged supplemental tube feedings have been shown to be at risk for developing behavioral feeding disorders.[21–23] These children may benefit from oral stimulation, which would reduce feeding difficulties and result in a more pleasurable feeding experience for both child and caregiver. It has been noted that chronically ill children, especially those who are tracheostomized, do demonstrate a higher risk for developing behavioral feeding difficulties as a result of their chronic illnesses. If the children are unable to consume their required caloric intake, "force feeding" may result and may further contribute to behavioral problems.

Other factors contributing to the development of behavioral feeding problems may be related to multiple caregivers using inconsistent approaches to mealtime. Periods of hospitalization, nursing time constraints, rigid scheduling, and frequent distractions may also interfere with children's successful feeding experiences.

•   •   •

With improvements in medical technology, a unique population of infants and young children has evolved. These infants and children require tracheostomy placement throughout their childhood. Therefore it is important for habilitative care to be initiated at an early age to maximize all areas of development, including speech, language, and voice. In addition, earlier identification of developmental delay may impact the child's overall maturational progress.

Speech and language intervention may be important to approximate articulatory movements necessary for later speech development and to provide augmentative/ alternative communication for children. Through the development of an expressive communication system during the period of cannulation, communicative frustration can be reduced. Early oral feeding experiences should also be provided for infants and children with tracheostomies to decrease the risk of severe feeding difficulties and the emergence of behavioral feeding problems. Improvements in oral feeding experiences during the period of cannulation have been helpful in decreasing long-term feeding difficulties commonly seen in this unique population. Management of children with long-term tracheostomies is a complex process that requires careful coordination and consistent follow-up in the areas of communication and feeding.

REFERENCES

1. Ross GS: Language functioning and speech development of six children receiving tracheostomy in infancy. *J Commun Dis* 1982,15:95.

2. Simon BM, Fowler SM, Handler SD: Communication development in young children with long-term tracheostomies: Preliminary report. *Int J Pediatr Otorhinolaryngol* 1983;6:37.

3. Bowman SA, Shanks JC, Manion MW: Effect of prolonged nasotracheal intubation on communication. *J Speech Dis* 1972;37:403.

4. Kaslon KW, Grabo DE, Ruben R: Voice, speech and language habilitation in young children without laryngeal function. *Arch Otolaryngol* 1978;104:737.

5. Tucker HA, Rusnov M, Cohen L: Speech development in aphonic children. *Laryngoscope* 1982;92:566.

6. Handler SD, Simon BM, Fowler S: Speech and the child with a long-term tracheostomy: The problem and otolaryngologist's role. *Trans Pa Acad Ophthalmol Otolaryngol* 1983;36:67.

7. Passy V: Passy-Muir tracheostomy speaking valve. *Otolaryngol Head Neck Surg* 1986;95:247.

8. Wetmore RF, Handler SD, Potsic WP: Pediatric tracheostomy: Experience during the past decade. *Ann Otol Rhinol Laryngol* 1982;91:628.

9. English ST, Prutting CA: Teaching American sign language to a normally hearing infant with tracheostenosis. *Clin Pediatr* 1975;14:1141.

10. Simon BM, Handler SD: The speech pathologist and management of children with tracheostomies. *J Otolaryngol* 1981;10:440.

11. Harlor M: Communication strategies for a child having total laryngeal stenosis: A case report. *J Pa Speech Lang Hear Assoc* 1983;16:2.

12. Levy SD, Fowler SM, Trachtenberg S, et al: Interdisciplinary rehabilitative team management for long-term hospitalized children. *Abstr Dev Med Child Neurol* 1986;28:114–115.

13. Fowler SM, Simon BM, Handler SD: Communication development in children, in Myers EN, Stool SE, Johnson JT, eds: *Tracheostomy.* New York, Churchill Livingstone, 1985.

14. Dinwiddie R, Mellor DH, Donaldson SHC, et al: Quality of survival after artificial ventilation of the newborn. *Arch Dis Child* 1974;49:703.

15. Ziegler MM, Shaw D, Goldberg AI, et al: Sequelae of prolonged ventilatory support for pediatric surgical patients. *J Pediatr Surg* 1979;14:768.

16. Kaslon KW, Stein RE: Chronic pediatric tracheostomy: Assessment and implications for habilitation of voice, speech and language in young children. *Int J Pediatr Otorhinolaryngology* 1985;9:165.

17. Singer LT, Wood R, Lambert S: Developmental follow-up of long-term infant tracheostomy: A preliminary report. *Dev Behav Pediatr* 1985;6:132.

18. Morris SE: The normal acquisition of oral feeding skills: Implications for assessment and treatment. New York, Therapeutic Media, 1982.

19. McGowan JS, Geyer LA: Videofluoroscopy: A multidisciplinary model for evaluating swallowing dysfunction in children. *Abstr Dev Med Child Neurol* 1986;28:29–30.

20. Bernbaum JC, Pereira G, Watkins JB, et al: Nonnutritive sucking during gavage feeding enhances growth and maturation in premature infants. *Pediatrics* 1983;71:41.

21. Illingworth RS, Lister J: The critical or sensitive period, with special reference to certain feeding problems in infants and children. *Pediatrics* 1964;65:839.

22. DiScipio WJ, Kaslon K, Ruben RJ: Traumatically acquired conditioned dysphagia in children. *Ann Otol Rhinol Laryngol* 1978;87:509.

23. Palmer S, Thompson RJ Jr, Linsheld TR: Applied behavior analysis in the treatment of childhood feeding problems. *Dev Med Child Neurol* 1975;17:333.

Early language intervention: When, why, how?

Rachel E. Stark, PhD
Department Head
Audiology and Speech Sciences
Purdue University
West Lafayette, Indiana

THE TITLE of this article suggests a riddle. All good riddles have a simple but highly satisfactory answer that is usually not obvious to any but the most insightful individual. Yet as soon as the answer is given, it is seen as right and inevitable by all. No such clear answers have emerged in the case of early language intervention. Indeed, there are differences of opinion among those who have the most experience and authority in the relevant fields of speech–language pathology, developmental psychology, and special education. However, with the advent of Public Law 99-457, which mandates the provision of appropriate educational and related services for preschool handicapped and at-risk children (0 to 5 years), it is important to resolve such differences and to arrive at clear guidelines for language intervention with preschool children, including infants and toddlers.

The first question that must be addressed is "Why early language intervention?" The arguments usually offered in relation to this question have to do with the improved effectiveness of intervention that is provided earlier in life as compared with later.[1] Early intervention, it is claimed, may take advantage of sensitive periods of development during which the central nervous system has the highest potential for growth and significant plasticity. Evidence for this claim, first put forth by Lenneberg,[2] has come from a number of studies. Vargha-Khadem et al[3] have shown that children with unilateral cortical lesions are most likely to show language recovery if the neurologic lesion is sustained before rather than after 5 years of age. In the early 1960s Whetnall and Fry[4] showed that children with mild-to-moderate hearing impairments who were not given appropriate hearing aids and language instruction in the preschool and early school years failed to acquire spoken language, although they had the potential to do so. Intervention provided for the first time in later school years was ineffective in reversing this unfortunate outcome.

Early intervention programs, such as Head Start, which have provided enriched environments to disadvantaged children, have almost always been reported as yielding immediate short-term gains in linguistic and cognitive development. Ramey and Haskins[5] have also pointed out, however, that these gains tend to "wash out" once the graduates of intervention programs enter grade school. Early intervention appears to be least effective when the child is not provided continued enrichment in grade school but is returned to an impoverished environment. This may not be entirely surprising. Why should children in grade school classes,

This article was supported by NIH grant #HD11970 and by Maternal and Child Health grant #MC-R-240447.

Inf Young Children 1989; 1(4): 44–53

where instruction must be targeted toward the majority of children who have not received early enrichment, be expected to solve new problems in language learning without continued modeling and examples? In spite of this disappointing outcome, longitudinal studies such as that of Seitz et al[6] have suggested that disadvantaged children do benefit in the long term from early intervention. They are less likely than their fellow students who did not receive intervention to repeat grades and to drop out of school in their early to midteens.

There are few studies of the effectiveness of language intervention among preschool children with neurologic lesions. Clearly, however, the inability to understand or to communicate as a result of head trauma or cerebral palsy, for example, will inhibit learning and intellectual development and should be addressed with intervention before such effects appear.

When should early language intervention begin? Some professionals believe that language intervention should not be provided until the child actually begins to speak. If this belief were adopted generally, high-risk infants (eg, ventilator-dependent infants in hospital care) would receive no language stimulation, and severely cerebral-palsied preschool children would be given no means to communicate. Other professionals recommend waiting until 2 or 2½ years of age before deciding that the nonspeaking child is not going to "talk on his or her own" and needs language intervention. This principle does not take account of such risk factors as prematurity, low socioeconomic status, and neurologic deficits, among others.

Factors to consider are the following:

- Is the child at risk, based on medical and family history factors ? If so, his or her language development should be monitored regularly.
- Is the child likely to experience speech and language deprivation because of socioeconomic factors or because of deafness in his or her parents? If so, every effort should be made to provide, or to help the parents provide, language stimulation in the home.
- Is a congenital anomaly present that is known to be associated with speech and language deficits (eg, cleft palate or hearing loss in the child)? If so, baseline prespeech measures should be obtained regularly in the first years of life and language intervention provided as appropriate.

Even when no risk factors or predisposing conditions are present, it is important that health-related professionals have some guidelines for deciding when to refer a nonspeaking preschool child to the speech–language pathologist or audiologist. How are late-normal, language-delayed, and severely language-impaired children to be differentiated in the first two years of life? They may be indistinguishable on the basis of observations made in a physician's office or even of parental report. It is essential to take into consideration known risk factors and the child's level of performance in prelinguistic skills in addition to the failure to acquire the language milestones normally appearing at 18 to 24 months of age.

Consider, for example, the hypothetical data shown in Fig 1. The linguistic units shown on the vertical axis could be speech sounds, words, sentences, or phrases. They are plotted against hypothetical age increments shown on the horizontal axis. The learning curve labeled as "high normal" in this figure initially shows a typical slow rate of learning followed by accelerated learning in the midportion, and then a subsequent leveling off. The curve labeled "low normal" represents the learning of a "late starter" who nevertheless has a normal potential and eventually catches up with his or her peers. The two curves on the far right illustrate the progress of the language-delayed child who continues to show a slower-than-normal rate of learning with little acceleration and whose learning may level off earlier (ie, at a lower level of achievement than for the normal child) and of the severely language-impaired child whose learning is even slower and more severely curtailed than for the language-delayed child.

Fig 1 illustrates the fact that some children, who later show normal language acquisition, may still be delayed in the onset of early language milestones. This delay in onset may be attributable to the fact that young children show a variety of cognitive and learning styles and strategies in their development of language. It has been suggested that in some cases a child's strategies are not compatible with the interactive style of the mother. In such a case the child may suffer at least a temporary delay in language acquisition.[7]

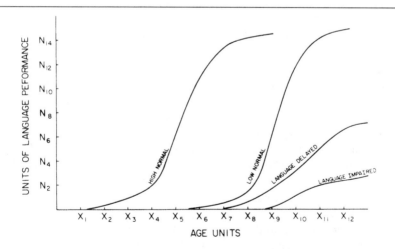

Fig 1. Idealized function representing the learning curve with respect to acquisition of hypothetical units of language by four groups of children. Reprinted with permission from Stark RE, Mellits ED, Tallal P: Behavioral attributes of speech and language disorders, in Ludlow CL and Cooper JA (eds): *Genetic Aspects of Speech and Language Disorders.* New York, Academic Press, 1983, p. 39.

Individual differences in language acquisition could also reflect differences with respect to the development of language-related skills (eg, speech discrimination, auditory sequencing, auditory memory, oral–motor coordination, sequencing of the movements for speech, or subtle representational abilities). Mild delays with respect to these abilities could give rise to a marked but temporary delay in language acquisition. Once the affected language-related skill attains a certain threshold level, it could be that the child suddenly begins to understand the nature and use of language more clearly, with a consequent integration of skills and acceleration of language development.[8]

The language-delayed child may show more severe delays in the acquisition of one or more language-related (perceptual–motor) skills than the normal "late starter." This child also may develop language-learning strategies that are not compatible with the interactive styles of his or her teachers or family members. He or she may fail to integrate certain aspects of language until much later than the "low-normal" child, may continue to develop language at a slower-than-normal rate, and, as a result, may experience difficulty with reading and academic work in later elementary school grades. The child who is severely language impaired may present more severe deficits in perceptual–motor or cognitive abilities or deficits across a greater number of abilities. His or her deficits may extend to social interaction and may be based on significant neurologic impairment instead of maturational lags.

Screening tools such as the Early Language Milestone Scale developed by Coplan[9] or the Clinical Linguistic and Auditory Milestone Scale developed by Capute and his colleague[10] are useful for the purpose of initial identification of children at risk for language delay or severe language impairment. The speech–language pathologist should use more comprehensive instruments, such as the Preschool Language Scale[11] or the Sequenced Inventory of Communication Development[12] in the speech and language evaluation of the child who fails such screening tests. Descriptive data that are based on the work of Oller,[13] Stark,[14] Stark et al,[15] and Netsell[16] provide a means of assessing the level of prelinguistic development that the nonspeaking preschool child has attained. Proposed levels of speech production based on studies of over 100 normal infants, for example, are shown in Appendix A. Such information is important not only for deciding on whether intervention is needed but also, if it is recommended, for deciding at what point it should begin.

In summary, referral to the speech–language pathologist, audiologist, or psychologist for evaluation and possible intervention should be made for the infant who

- is at high risk for language delay because of family or medical history factors;
- is clearly delayed in acquiring prespeech production milestones;

- does not respond normally to the speech of others;
- shows atypical language learning curves or significant deficits in language-related skills; and
- shows signs of a cognitive delay or deficit.

The decision may then be made as to whether to monitor progress, to provide natural language stimulation, or to recommend diagnostic therapy or intervention.

How should language intervention be provided? The answer to this question depends on the careful determination of (1) the nature of the child's language impairment and (2) the degree of impairment. For example, if the child's language impairment appears to be relatively mild and if few risk factors appear to be involved, then a nonspecific language stimulation program may be the most appropriate treatment. This program may be provided in a regular preschool setting or in an integrated preschool. The members of the child's immediate family should be included in the day-to-day planning for intervention and should be shown how to extend the language stimulation into everyday activities in the home.

If the child's language is severely impaired or is developing in an unusual way, then a more specific treatment program must be designed to meet the child's needs. In-depth evaluation of the risk factors and the child's level of performance on prespeech measures and measures of component (language-related) skills (eg, speech perception, speech production, and vocal communication) should be employed for this purpose. Otherwise, different approaches and different philosophies may conflict with one another.

Two of the most frequently advocated approaches are described below.

- One approach is based on an established developmental sequence for a particular set of skills (eg, those involved in language development and in cognitive development).
- Another approach is based on an estimate of functional skills required in a particular environment and on behavior modification techniques designed to yield these requisite skills.

Are both approaches valid ones, depending on the child's level of functioning and his or her specific needs? If so, how is the clinician to make a reasonable choice of approach in a given child's case? It may be of value to examine a particular problem area in considering such alternatives, namely that of pragmatic functioning.

A number of developmental sequences have been proposed for the acquisition of communication behaviors in infants, notably those of Halliday,[17] Dunst,[18] Dore,[19] Dale et al,[20] and Stark et al.[21] Appendix B shows levels of vocalization behavior according to communicative context as proposed by Stark et al.[21] The estimated age of acquisition of each of these levels is derived from a home-based study of 50 normal infants. It will be observed that many of the terms employed are those proposed by Halliday.[17] Halliday's subject, however, was studied from 6 to 18 months of age. In the study by Stark et al,[21] terms were added that were considered appropriate for younger infants (0 to 6 months). All terms were defined or described in terms of the context of vocal behavior. The descriptions or definitions were made up of nonvocal behaviors, such as facial expression, gesture, or other movements that accompany vocalization, context (eg, feeding), and the responses of adults interacting with the child.

It will also be observed that the earliest category (reflexive) is the same as that employed in the first level in Appendix A, in which speech–motor aspects of infant vocalizations are described. The duplication of terms reflects the close correspondence between the acoustic (physical) aspects and articulatory (speech movement) features of sounds produced by infants of 0 to 2 months of age and their communicative context.

Information of the kind shown in Appendix B has already proved useful in determining delays in social communicative functioning in developmentally disabled children (eg, children whose ability to produce the articulatory movements and sounds of speech is relatively good but who may be using speech sounds in a socially aberrant manner). At one time it was suggested to colleagues that this preliminary scale might be useful in evaluating the vocal communicative behavior of children with severe cerebral palsy. Yet in spite of a genuine interest in the approach, these colleagues instead developed "scripts" (eg, relating to a family picnic) that were designed to elicit a variety of communicative behaviors from children with severe sensorimotor disabilities. Because it was important to elicit during assessment any kind of communicative behavior available to the child (eg, facial expression, laughter, directed gaze, pointing response, as well as vocalization), pretend activities of high interest to children had to be created, not merely contexts in which the child might vocalize. Here present function was seen as more important than developmental information about one particular aspect of social communication (vocalization).

It is the author's view that in language intervention the development of abilities that are most delayed should be facilitated or taught directly. To do so one must determine the level the child has already attained in the most affected (weakest) area. If one attempts to begin treatment at a higher level, progress may be inhibited. Scales to be developed from the information summarized in Appendices A and B will be important for this purpose. Every effort should be made to integrate the more slowly developing skills with those that are more advanced. The process of integration must begin at the level the child has attained in his or her weakest area.[8] For example, if a child's comprehension of language, and in particular his or her grasp of word meanings, is severely delayed, it will not be profitable to teach him or her to produce words and sentences far above his or her level of comprehension. Approaches of this kind are sometimes undertaken in treating children whose expressive language abilities already exceed their receptive language abilities. They merely serve to exacerbate the child's problem. Instead of teaching him or her to say "That's a Thanksgiving turkey. It is orange and yellow," it may be more productive for him or her to learn to say, "I wanna go play" or "I wanna push (eg, the elevator button)" in meaningful and productive exchanges.

A developmentally based approach may not work as well, however, with severely to profoundly handicapped children, especially those who have multiple handicaps (eg, the cerebral-palsied children with augmentative/alternative communication systems whose interactive capabilities were assessed by means of "scripts"). Consider also the profoundly handicapped 13-year-old who pushes food and drink away vigorously when he or she does not want it, upsetting the contents of cup and plate. Such behavior might be typical of a normal 6- to 9-month-old infant. If, however, it were possible to teach this 13-year-old to produce a verbal regulatory response, the word "No!," then his or her behavior might be more acceptable in a mainstreamed activity. Thus he or she might be able to benefit from experience in a greater variety of settings. It would not be reasonable to insist that this child first learn to vocalize during activities such as banging or mouthing objects (an earlier level in the proposed scale shown in Appendix D). He or she may, in fact, have shown these behaviors at an earlier period in his or her life. Such developmentally appropriate behaviors are not always maintained in children who remain for a long time at the same cognitive or prelinguistic level.

It is the author's view that the developmental levels that a language-impaired child has attained across a number of areas (speech perception, speech production, receptive language, expressive language, cognitive [representational] abilities) should be taken into account in designing intervention. However, in the case of a child with multiple handicaps, especially where one or more handicaps are severe to profound, it may be more important to examine the child's functional needs and the demands of his or her environment. Behavioral strategies may then be employed to improve his or her functioning, thus circumventing developmental problems. Both approaches, the developmental and the behavioral, may be of value, however; and both should be considered even for children with single handicaps of great severity and for those with multiple handicaps.

•   •   •

In summary, the evidence obtained thus far suggests that early language intervention is effective if it is designed to meet the needs of the individual child. The decisions when to intervene and how best to intervene depend on careful assessment of the risk factors, predisposing conditions, the child's pattern of deficits, and the severity of his or her language impairment. Developmental information with respect to the child's prespeech perception and production of sounds and his or her social communicative behavior should be obtained as well as an estimate of his or her cognitive abilities. However, intervention may need, in cases of severe and multiple handicaps, to address the child's functional needs directly and by means of behavior modification strategies. Such decisions should always be made in cooperation with the child's family members.

REFERENCES

1. Johnston RB, Magrab PR: *Developmental Disorders: Assessment, Treatment, Education.* Baltimore, University Park Press, 1976.
2. Lenneberg E: *Biological Foundations of Language.* New York, Wiley, 1967.
3. Vargha-Khadem F, O'Gorman AM, Walters GV: Aphasia and handedness in relation to hemispheric side, age at injury and severity of cerebral lesion during childhood. *Brain* 1985;108:677–696.
4. Whetnall E, Fry DB: *The Deaf Child.* Springfield, Ill, Charles C Thomas, 1964.
5. Ramey CT, Haskins R: The causes and treatment of school failure: Insights from the Carolina Abecedarian Project, in Begab MJ, Haywood HC, Garver HL (eds): *Psychosocial Influences in Retarded Performance: Vol II.* Baltimore, University Park Press, 1981, pp 89–112.
6. Seitz V, Apfel NH, Rosenbaum LK: Projects head start and follow through: A longitudinal evaluation of adolescents, in Begab MJ, Haywood HC, Garber HL (eds): *Psychosocial Influences in Retarded Performance: Vol II.* Baltimore, University Park Press, 1981, pp 17–28.
7. Nelson K: Structure and strategy in learning to talk. *Monographs of the Society for Research in Child Development* 1973;38:1–2, Serial #149.
8. Stark RE: Implications for clinical management, in Stark RE, Tallal P, McCauley RJ (eds): *Language, Speech and Reading Disorders in Children: Neuropsychological Studies.* San Diego, College-Hill Press, 1988, pp 169–180.
9. Coplan J: *The Early Language Milestone Scale.* Tulsa, Okla, Modern Education, 1983.
10. Capute AJ, Accardo PJ: Linguistic and auditory milestones during the first two years of life. *Clin Pediatr* 1978;17:847–853.
11. Zimmerman IL, Steiner VG, Pond RE: *Preschool Language Scale.* Columbus, Oh, Charles E. Merrill, 1979.
12. Hedrick DL, Prather EM, Tobin AR: *Sequenced Inventory of Communication Development.* Seattle, Wash, University of Washington Press, 1975.
13. Oller DK: The emergence of the sounds of speech in infancy, in Yenikomshian G, Ferguson C, Kavanagh J (eds): *Child Phonology Vol I: Production.* New York, Academic Press, 1980, pp 93–112.
14. Stark RE: Prespeech segmental feature development, in Fletcher P, Garman M (eds): *Studies in Language Acquisition,* rev ed. Cambridge, England, Cambridge University Press, 1986, pp 149–173.
15. Stark RE, Ansel BM, Bond J: Are prelinguistic abilities predictive of learning disability?, in Masland MA, Masland RL (eds): *Preschool Prevention of Reading Failure.* Parkton, Md, York Press, 1988.
16. Netsell R: The acquisition of speech motor control: A perspective with directions for research, in Stark RE (ed): *Language Behavior in Infancy and Early Childhood.* New York, Elsevier/North Holland, 1981, pp 127–156.

17. Halliday MAK: *Learning How To Mean: Explorations in the Functions of Language.* London, Edward Arnold, 1973.

18. Dunst C: A cognitive-social approach for assessment of early nonverbal communicative behavior. *J Child Commun Dis* 1978;2:110–123.

19. Dore J: Holophrases, speech acts and language universals. *J Child Lang* 1975;2:21–40.

20. Dale PS, Cook N, Goldstein H: Pragmatics and symbolic play: A study in language and cognitive development. Paper presented at the Biennial Meeting of the Society for Research in Child Development, 1978.

21. Stark RE, Bernstein LE, Demorest ME: Assessment of vocal communication in young children. *ASHA* 1983;25:56.

Appendix A

Levels of speech/motor/skill attained by the infant at different age levels

Level	Brief description	Anticipated age of onset
1. Reflexive	Sustained crying Fasting sounds Vegetative sounds Quasiresonant nucleus (ie, small grunt) Fully resonant nucleus (ie, a sound produced with open mouth that is harsh, not vowel-like)	0–2 months

2. Control of
    phonation
	Single vowel
	Combination of vowel with trill, friction
	    consonant, or nasal murmur
	Syllabic nasal consonant (eg, /m/)
	Chuckle
	Sustained laughter
		2–4 months

3 and 4.
    Expansion:
    Control of
    articulation
    and pitch
	Prolonged inspiratory sounds
	Squeal
	Series of vowels
	Vowels with glide
	Isolated prolonged consonant
	Series of isolated consonants
	Marginal babbling
		5–6 months

5. Babbling:
    Syllable
    production
	Consonant-vowel (CV) syllable
	Reduplicated (repeated) CV syllable series
	Simple, nonreduplicated CV syllable series
	Yell
		7–9 months

continues

Level	Brief description	Anticipated age of onset
6 and 7. New syllable types and expressive jargon	Vowels /i/ as in "see" and /u/ as in "too"	10–18 months
	Other rounded vowels (eg, /o/ as in "toe")	
	Diphthongs (eg, /au/ as in "out")	
	Syllables other than CV	
	Whisper	
	More complex nonreduplicated syllable series	
	Jargon	

Appendix B

Levels of vocalization behavior in the normal infant according to the communicative context or communicative intent with which they are produced

Level	Brief description of context	Anticipated age of onset
	Sounds according to context	
1. Reflexive	Cry	0–2 months
	Discomfort	
	Small grunts	
	Vegetative	
2. Reactive	Comfort:	2–4 months
	In response to persons	
	In response to objects	
	Neutral:	
	In response to persons	
	In response to objects	
	Chuckle	
	Laughter	
3. Activity	Visual attention to objects	4–6 months
	Objects in mouth	
	Manipulation of objects (eg, banging, shaking)	
	Locomotion	
	Other movement	
1. Personal	*Sounds according to intent*	7–9 months
	Self-conscious expressions of feeling	
	Showing off	

continues

Level	Brief description of context	Anticipated age of onset
2. Instrumental/ regulatory	Requesting object Requesting activity Rejecting object Rejecting activity	9–12 months
3. Interactional	Greetings Ritual exchanges Imitation of adult Commenting on objects Commenting on activity Noticing objects	12–15 months
4. Heuristic/ imaginative and other	Onomatopoeic sounds (eg, animal and car noises) Agreement ("Yes") Disagreement ("No") Naming Requesting names Imaginative play Commenting on appearance/disappearance of objects	16–24 months

Developmental intervention with the chronically ill infant

Toby Long, MA, PT
Director, Division of Physical Therapy

Kathy Katz, PhD
Director, Division of Psychology

Judith Pokorni, PhD
Co-director, Division of Special
  Education
Georgetown University Child
  Development Center
Washington, DC

TECHNOLOGICAL advances in neonatal care have resulted in dramatically increased survival rates for low-birthweight premature infants and other infants with major medical complications.[1] While the prognosis for no major handicapping condition has increased for most nursery survivors, the estimate of major handicap for the smallest survivors is about 30%.[2] These infants often remain medically fragile because of respiratory compromise, tracheostomies, gastrostomy tubes, seizure disorders, and other severe neurologic damage.

The Georgetown University Child Development Center has provided developmental follow-up of infants discharged from the neonatal intensive care unit (NICU) of Georgetown University Hospital for the past ten years. Developmental evaluations are performed on a regular basis during the first two years of life. In addition to evaluations, the physical and occupational therapists of the Child Development Center began providing direct treatment to the most vulnerable infants in the nursery. Although infants were being identified early as needing developmental support, many had no access to community-based programs because of significant medical needs that resulted in long hospital stays, multiple rehospitalizations, or numerous outpatient medical services.

Concern for this very special group of infants led to the development of the Chronically Ill Infant Intervention (CIII) Project, which received funding in 1985 as a Handicapped Children's Early Education Program from the U.S. Department of Education, Office of Special Education Programs. The purpose of the project is twofold. The first purpose is to provide continuity of developmental support to chronically ill and medically fragile infants. This is initiated in the NICU and is carried through to discharge to home or to the pediatric intensive care unit (PICU). The support is continued in the event of readmission to the hospital. The second purpose is to provide support and training to parents in understanding the developmental needs of their chronically ill and medically fragile infant.

The authors would like to acknowledge Dani LeMense and Laura Norden for designing the artwork for this article. This project was supported by a grant from the U.S. Department of Education, Office of Special Education Programs grant #G008530081.

Inf Young Children 1989; 1(4): 78–88
© 1989 Aspen Publishers, Inc.

THE PROJECT

The CIII Project consists of three interrelated components: (1) the NICU phase, (2) the home-based phase, and (3) the PICU phase. The design of each phase and the intervention strategies used are based on a family-centered approach to the care of at-risk and handicapped infants. The family-centered approach is based on the belief that needs of the child and the family as a whole are interrelated. As a result, the CIII Project works collaboratively with the family during each phase in evolving an intervention plan that provides a level of involvement with which they feel comfortable.

THE TEAM

The project team consists of a pediatric psychologist who serves as the project director, a special educator, a physical therapist, and a pediatric nurse practitioner. The team works together to form a plan that interfaces with the needs of the family. Each family is assigned a case manager from among the project team. This person remains the primary contact person for the family. The boxed material entitled "Case Manager Responsibilities" outlines the responsibilities of the case manager during each phase of the project.

Case Manager Responsibilities

NICU component
Liaison with hospital staff:
  primary nurses
  social worker
  neonatologists
Assist in discharge planning
Family support:
  enroll families
  maintain ongoing communication
Child intervention:
  attend at weekly CIII staffing
  coordinate developmental recommendations
Home-based component
Liaison with medical and nursing personnel:
  primary pediatrician
  specialty clinics
  visiting and home-care nurses
Family support:
  identify family needs

  attend family-focused interview
  maintain regular contact
  assist in accessing services
Child intervention:
  attend at weekly CIII staffing
  coordinate developmental plan
PICU component
Liaison with hospital staff:
  primary nurses
  social worker
  pediatricians
Family support:
  identify family needs
  maintain ongoing communication
Child intervention:
  attend PICU child life rounds
  coordinate developmental plan
  assist in discharge planning

Disciplinary roles are broken down in a more traditional format related to the expertise of the team member. The psychologist provides consultation to the team and to the families regarding psychosocial and behavioral issues. As project director, the psychologist also attends the weekly social service rounds held in the special care nursery. There he or she identifies families who are appropriate for the project. Feedback is also provided to the medical staff at this time on the needs of the families already enrolled in the project.

The special educator develops caregiving recommendations for the family and NICU staff based on observations of the infant's behavioral responses while in the nursery. He or she provides direct educational activities as the infant matures and is available for interaction.

A therapeutic positioning plan is designed and carried out by the physical therapist. As the infant is able to tolerate handling, the therapist initiates a program of direct treatment based on neurodevelopmental principles.

A major focus for the project nurse practitioner is to help the family coordinate discharge planning and to ensure that the family is linked with the appropriate community-based health care services.

THE POPULATION

Thirty-four infants were enrolled in the project in the first year (17 intervention, 17 contrast). The project accepted the most vulnerable infants. During the first year of the project, three infants in the intervention group and two in the contrast group died. Infants were considered for enrollment if they met one or more of the following criteria:

- birthweight less than 1000 g,
- gestational age less than 28 weeks,
- length of stay more than three months,
- prolonged (more than six weeks) mechanical support,
- major central nervous system (CNS) insult such as intraventricular hemorrhage, or
- complex congenital anomalies that would require rehospitalization for correction.

Demographic profiles of both groups were similar. Mean birthweight was 1,345.1 g for the intervention group and 1,318.8 g for the contrast group. Mean gestational age was 29.1 and 29.4 weeks, respectively. Information regarding neonatal complications in both groups is listed in Table 1. The infants in each group were matched for medical complications, race, gender, and socioeconomic status. All families in the intervention group lived within a 30-mile radius of Georgetown University Hospital. The contrast group was made up of infants who met the selection criteria but who either were transferred back to a community hospital within

Table 1. Medical complications

Complication	Intervention	Contrast
Intraventricular hemorrage (IVH) (III, IV)	3	6
Periventricular leukomalacia	1	1
Hydrocephalus	2	1
Bronchopulmonary dysplasia	10	12
Retinopathy of prematurity	11	7
Congenital anomalies	2	2

the first few weeks of life or came from a family who resided outside the 30-mile radius.

PROGRAM COMPONENTS

Neonatal Intensive care unit component

Infants are enrolled in the CIII Project as soon as their health status suggests a good chance of immediate survival. At the time of enrollment, a case manager is linked with the family and continues in this capacity for the next two years. The CIII special educator conducts a structured behavioral observation of the infant using the Naturalistic Observation of Newborn Behavior.[3] This observation is designed to identify the individual infant's responses to environmental stimulation. Observations of the infant are made during a caregiving procedure. The behavioral responses of the infant to the caregiving are recorded and grouped according to autonomic, motor, state, and interaction systems.[4] Behaviors include stress signs, self-regulatory signs, and approach behaviors.[5] Patterns of behavioral responses are identified, are discussed with the infant's caregivers and family, and become the basis for developmental recommendations. Recommendations typically relate to decreasing stress, promoting state organization, and facilitating alert behavior. The boxed material, "Recommendations To Reduce Excessive Stimulation," lists some of the more common recommendations made.

The physical therapist performs a neuromotor evaluation using the Neonatal Neurobehavioral Examination (NNE).[6] The NNE provides information on reflex development, postural responses, muscle tone, and response to handling, taking into consideration the degree of prematurity of the infant. Following the evaluation, specific positioning and handling strategies are developed. Parents and caregivers are instructed in the appropriate techniques to meet the needs of individual infants. Figure 1 shows the positions preferred to increase flexion and a midline orientation of the extremities and head.

Recommendations To Reduce Excessive Stimulation

To reduce excess noise:
- Gently lower the head on the isolette mattress tray.
- Close portholes and isolette cabinets quietly.
- Eliminate finger tapping on isolettes.
- Discontinue the audible heart rate.
- Reduce talking over the isolette or across rooms.
- Eliminate radios or reduce their use to designated periods and confine music to calm, soothing variety.

To reduce bright lighting:
- Cover isolettes with blankets or filtering acetate.
- Adjust lighting to day/night cycles.

To reduce excess activity of the infant:
- Establish quiet times.
- Move less acute infants to a quiet area.
- Nest the baby with blanket rolls and swaddling.
- Provide finger rolls.
- Provide nonnutritive sucking.
- Feed in a quiet corner and minimize interaction.

Recommendations made by the educator and the physical therapist are formally written as a developmental care plan and are posted on the isolette and written in a communication book. The communication book is used by the CIII team, family, and medical staff as a means of sharing information about a particular infant. This has proven especially helpful for families who have difficulty visiting during week days.

The CIII nurse practitioner works closely with the NICU staff and the family in developing a discharge plan to ensure a smooth transition to home. Coordination of both medical and developmental services takes place through a process that begins weeks before the anticipated discharge. This includes assisting in the coordination of services provided by agencies such as the Visiting Nurses Association, home nursing care agencies, and durable medical equipment suppliers.

The NICU component relies heavily on the facilitative model, working closely with the NICU staff members and relying on them to incorporate developmental recommendations into routine caregiving. Providing inservice training to the nursing staff was found to be extremely important to the effectiveness of this model.

The CIII team, in conjunction with a group of interested nurses, initiated a series of inservice presentations regarding the developmental needs of medically fragile infants and their families. The following topics were chosen based on the results of a needs assessment of the nursing staff conducted by the CIII team:

- the effects of the nursery environment on the infant and family,
- behavioral cues of the premature infant,
- parent–infant attachment in the special care nursery,
- therapeutic positioning and handling in the special care nursery,

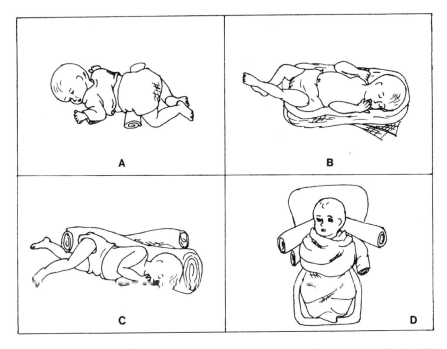

Fig 1. Therapeutic positions in prone (**A**), supine (**B**), and sidelying to promote flexion (**C**) and a midline orientation of extremities and head (**D**).

- development in the first year—full-term *v* preterm,
- the importance of developmental follow up,
- the physician's role in developmental intervention,
- forming a developmental committee, and
- enhancing the parental role as caregiver.

Several one-hour inservice sessions were scheduled, and reading material was provided in the nurses' lounge and at the nurses' station. The most effective vehicle for providing information to the nurses proved to be a two-day developmental conference organized by the nursing staff with assistance from the CIII team. Nursing administration supported this conference by providing release time for nurses to attend.

The nursing staff was also instrumental in incorporating an introduction to developmental intervention as part of the orientation program for NICU. In this way nurses who are beginning work in the NICU have a basic awareness of such areas as effects of the NICU environment on infants and positioning and handling of infants. As a result of the collaboration between nurses and the CIII team, both preservice and inservice training now include a focus on developmental intervention in the NICU.

Home intervention component

Because the CIII infant's health status typically precludes immediate enrollment into a community-based infant intervention program, the family receives CIII home-based intervention services on discharge to home. The family's CIII case manager continues to bear primary responsibility for working with the family to coordinate services. Approximately two weeks after discharge, the case manager arranges a planning meeting with the family, referred to as a "family-focused interview."[6,7] This meeting is held in the family's home, and all family members are invited to attend. The psychologist and case manager of the CIII team are also present. The goal of the interview is to assist the family in defining a plan of action for caring for the special needs of the infant at home and determining other family needs that may affect the care of the infant. At this meeting, the Individualized Family Support Plan (IFSP) is developed, emphasizing the goals and needs of the family.

Typically a family receives intensive support from the CIII nurse during the first few weeks at home. Many of the infants in the program are discharged on apnea monitors, oxygen support, and nasogastric feeding. Parents receive training and support from the nurse in management of the infant to ease the transition from the highly supportive NICU environment to home. As the infant's medical condition stabilizes and the family becomes more comfortable with the care of the infant, nursing visits decrease. Most families do not require CIII nursing services after the first four months at home. In addition to the technological support and training, the nurse provides information and assistance regarding feeding, sleeping, and other infant care issues that may be difficult for the family to manage due to the medical fragility of the infant.

Special education services and physical therapy interventions are designed according to the needs of the infant. Often a weekly visit is provided by each specialist initially with services gradually decreasing as the child progresses. As the infant becomes medically stable, plans are made for integration into community-based intervention programs. The CIII team uses a holistic approach to the treatment of infants based on a neurodevelopmental philosophy. Because the team is committed to the philosophy that parents are the primary caregivers, parents are integral participants during each visit. Direct instruction in appropriate activities is provided and suggestions are left with the family in the communication book. This proves especially helpful for working parents whose infant is seen by the CIII team in a babysitting or home nursing care situation.

During each home visit, documentation of the concerns of both parents and CIII staff is made. Concerns include both developmental needs of the child and family needs. A content analysis of the documentation over the first 18 months was conducted to assess possible trends in developmental concerns. Ten areas of concern were clustered in the following four areas: education, motor, caregiving, and parent support.

The education cluster includes cognitive, speech–language, social–emotional, and behavioral issues. The motor cluster consists of skills related to fine and gross motor development and neuromotor maturation. Caregiving includes concerns related to feeding, sleeping, health, and physiologic equilibrium. The emotional needs of the family are included in the parent support cluster.

Concerns noted at each visit were coded for level of severity. A four-point scoring system was used, with 0 = no concern; 1 = minimal concern, requiring monitoring through regular developmental clinic visits, parent group meetings, developmental play groups, and telephone calls; 2 = moderate concern, requiring regular follow-up through home visitation (biweekly or monthly) with caregiving or activity suggestions to parents, and 3 = severe concern, requiring acute, ongoing, direct intervention on a weekly basis.

An analysis of the data[8] using Friedman's two-way analysis of variance by rank (Table 2) indicated several trends.[9] The need for motor intervention remained constant over the first 18 months. Caregiving concerns and parental support needs

---

Table 2. Determining changes in family needs, 0–18 months ($N = 14$)

Need	Charge
Parent support	$\chi^2 = 7.8^*$
Motor	$\chi^2 = 4.2$
Education	$\chi^2 = 21.0^\dagger$
Cognition	$\chi^2 = 14.0^\ddagger$
Speech and language	$\chi^2 = 14.5^\ddagger$
Social and emotional	$\chi^2 = 3.0$
Behavioral	$\chi^2 = 4.0$
Caregiving	$\chi^2 = 8.2^*$
Feeding	$\chi^2 = 1.7$
Sleeping	$\chi^2 = 1.8$
Health	$\chi^2 = 10.9^\S$
Physiological equilibrium	$\chi^2 = 6.3^*$

df = 3
* $p < .05$
† $p < .001$
‡ $p < .01$
§ $p < .02$

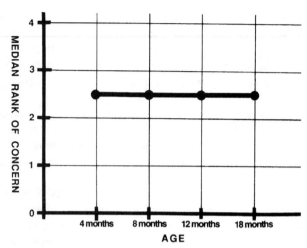

Fig 2. Trends in intervention needs over time: Motor concerns.

decreased over time, and educational needs, especially language, increased significantly during the first 18 months. Figs 2 through 5 show the trends determined by this analysis. The services provided by the CIII intervention team reflect these trends.

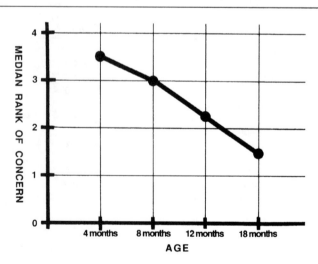

Fig 3. Trends in intervention needs over time: Caregiving concerns.

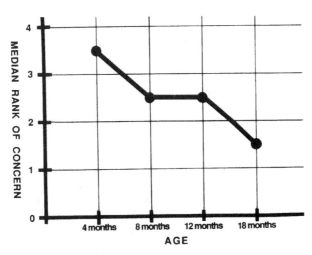

Fig 4. Trends in intervention needs over time: Parent support concerns.

During the home-based phase, a major thrust is to prepare the infant and family for transition into community-based services as soon as possible. Typically this transition occurs between 12 and 24 months. Services may include center-based intervention programs, home-based programs, individual therapy, or regular day

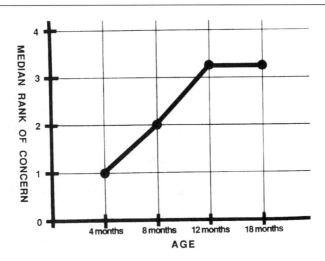

Fig 5. Trends in intervention needs over time: Education concerns.

care situations. Some children who are medically stable prior to 12 months and have a significant handicap are transitioned into an intensive daily intervention program .

Pediatric intensive care unit component

It was expected that some of the infants enrolled in the CIII Project would need hospitalization on the PICU directly from the NICU, or on rehospitalization from home. The infants who are transferred from the NICU to the PICU usually suffer from severe bronchopulmonary dysplasia or feeding intolerance and often remain on the unit for many months.

Infants requiring repeated surgical procedures, evaluation of failure to thrive, or treatment for upper respiratory infections are admitted to the special care unit of the PICU. During the infant's stay, the CIII team continues to provide needed services. The nurse and case manager provide support and information to the parents regarding the unit and any changes in medical management procedures. Intervention continues from the special educator and physical therapist as tolerated by the infant. For children who remain on the PICU for several months, educational and therapeutic services are provided two to three times per week for 30 to 60 minutes per visit. This is adjusted to the individual infant's needs and physical tolerance. The IFSP is updated on a regular basis to reflect the changing medical needs of the infant, the family situation, and the developmental status of the infant.

These three components—NICU, homebased intervention, and the PICU— form the structural framework of the CIII Project. Fig 6 provides a schematic of the project components.

•   •   •

The Chronically Ill Infant Intervention Project is designed to provide continuity in developmental services to medically fragile infants and their families. The intervention initiated in the NICU is based on the family-centered model of care. An interdisciplinary team of professionals provides ongoing developmental support addressing both family and infant needs.

The passage of Public Law 99-457 mandates the provision of service to this very special group of families in many states. For intervention to be effective, developmental specialists must be prepared to work collaboratively with medical personnel and families. The CIII Project has developed an intervention model that supports the family's role as primary caregiver and advocate for their infant.

Provision of services within a family-focused context requires a flexible service-delivery model. To meet the needs of the family, an intervention model must be adaptable to changes in those needs. Based on preliminary data of intervention

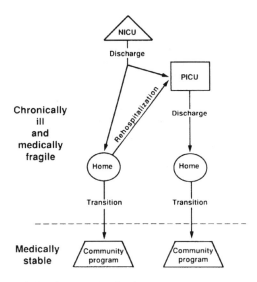

Fig 6. Chronically Ill Infant Intervention Project model.

needs over time, motor input should be made available to families throughout the first 18 months of life. During the first few months, there should be an emphasis on providing support and information regarding caregiving issues such as feeding, sleep patterns, and bathing. At about 12 months of age, more traditional educational concerns should be addressed. The experiences of the CIII team indicate that it is essential that interventionists be flexible to deal with both the developmental goals related to their own specialty area and the wide range of concerns that families may have about providing care to chronically ill and medically fragile infants.

REFERENCES

1. Bennett F, Robinson N, Sells C: Growth and development of infants weighing less than 800 grams at birth. *Pediatrics* 1983;17:319–323.

2. Hack M, Fanaroff A: Changes in the delivery room care of the extremely small infant (<750g): Effects on morbidity and outcome. *N Engl J Med* 1986;314:660–664.

3. Als H: *Manual for the Naturalistic Observation of Newborn Behavior (Preterm and Full Term Infants)*. Boston, Mass, Children's Hospital, 1984.

4. Als H: A synactive model of neonatal behavioral organization: Framework for the assessment of neurobehavioral development in the premature infant and for support of infants and parents in the neonatal intensive care environment. *Phys Occup Ther Pediatr* 1986;6:3–53.

5. Als H, Lawhorn G, Brown E, et al: Individualized behavioral and environmental care for the very low birthweight preterm infant at high risk for bronchopulmonary dysplasia: Neonatal intensive care unit and developmental outcome. *Pediatrics* 1986; 78:1123–1132.

6. Morgan A, Koch V, Lee V, et al: Neonatal neurobehavioral examination: A new instrument for quantitative analysis of neonatal neurological status. *Phys Ther* 1988;68:1352–1358.

7. Winton PJ, Bailey DB: The family-focused interview: A collaborative mechanism for family assessment and goal setting. *J Div Early Child* 1988;12:195–207.

8. Trends in intervention needs of a group of high-risk infants during the first 18 months. Paper presented at the National Center for Clinical Infant Programs, 5th Biennial National Training Institute, Washington, DC, Dec 6,1987.

9. Blalock HM: *Social Statistics*, ed 2. London, McGraw-Hill International, 1984.

Serving the young child with visual impairments: An overview of disability impact and intervention needs

Alana M. Zambone, PhD
National Consultant in Multiple
  Disabilities and Early Childhood
American Foundation for the Blind
New York, New York

IT IS anticipated that by 1990 approximately 20,000 children under the age of 5 years will have a visual impairment.[1] This number is particularly significant when one considers that it represents about two thirds of the total number of school-age children with visual impairments reported during the 1983–1984 academic year.[2] A visual impairment can be regarded as a "handicap of access" to the information and feedback that are necessary to learning.

Despite varying estimates of how much learning takes place via the visual system, it is generally assumed that "a greater quantity of information is gained in a shorter period of time through the use of the visual system than through any other single sense organ."[3(p86)] Given the importance of vision in development and learning, and the response of the visual system to training, a visual impairment can result in severe, if sometimes subtle, developmental delay and acquisition of secondary handicaps, particularly in the absence of early intervention. Thus the infant, toddler, or preschool-age child with a visual impairment is in need of services to ensure that the impact of the visual loss on development and learning is minimal and to ensure that the child is able to make maximum use of remaining vision.

The purpose of this article is to provide an overview of the impact of a visual impairment on development and learning. Critical components of intervention are discussed, and the roles of various team members in service delivery are briefly described.

COMMON VISUAL DISORDERS

There are a large number and variety of eye conditions found in young children who exhibit visual difficulties. Essentially problems in the visual system (ie, eye, optic nerve, or brain) affect the ability to see in one or more of five different categories of visual function:

1. Sending light to the retina—if one of the structures in the eye becomes damaged, as in development of cataracts (opacity of the lens), then light and images are not able to travel from the surface of the eye to the retina.
2. Focusing images on the retina—often, because of anomalies in the structures through which light passes (eg, an astigmatism or "wrinkle" in the cornea) or in the size and shape of the eye, images are not focused on the retina, resulting in conditions such as myopia (nearsightedness) or hyperopia (farsightedness).

Inf Young Children 1989; 2(2): 11–23

3. Transmission of nerve impulses to the brain— disorders of the retina (eg, the retinopathy of prematurity) or of the optic nerve (eg, optic nerve hypoplasia) may prevent images directed to the retina from being received and acted on by the retina and sent to the brain.

4. Processing of information received from the brain—damage to the visual cortex in the occipital lobes of the brain or severe generalized cerebral dysfunction resulting in significant intellectual deficits may also result in an inability of the brain to interpret visual information in a meaningful way. Often this type of impairment is given a generalized diagnostic label of "cortical blindness."

5. Coordination and direction of the eyes toward visual stimuli—defects in the muscles or in the structures of the eyes may interfere with the ability of the eyes to look at and focus on an image, or with their ability to do so together, as in strabismus. This can interfere with receiving, transmitting, or processing visual information accurately. Of equal or greater concern is the secondary condition of amblyopia, resulting from lack of use of one eye because of confusing images such as "double vision." With lack of use the eye eventually ceases to function.

The more common diagnoses in children with visual impairment include albinism, amblyopia, aniridia, cataracts, cortical blindness, diabetic retinopathy (juvenile diabetes), glaucoma, hyperopia, microphthalmia, myopia, nystagmus, optic atrophy, optic nerve hypoplasia, retinitis pigmentosa, retinopathy of prematurity, and strabismus. Many of these conditions are readily apparent through observation of the eye; all can be diagnosed through a medical examination. Those conditions that are not associated with outward abnormalities in the appearance of the eye, however, may not be diagnosed in the very young child or in the child with severe disabilities unless a specific referral for an eye examination is made. Thus it is important, particularly in the presence of attending conditions such as diabetes or cerebral palsy, that teachers and others in contact with the child carefully monitor response to visual stimulation so that examinations can be provided as needed.

Of the myriad of eye conditions seen in infants and toddlers with visual impairment, one condition, retinopathy of prematurity (ROP), formerly referred to as retrolental fibroplasia (RLF), has become one of the most common causes of childhood blindness in the United States today.[4-6] In the late 1940s and early 1950s blindness from RLF was considered to be epidemic. Changes in the concentration of oxygen in incubators nearly eradicated this condition.[7] With advancing medical technology during the 1970s and 1980s, however, increasing numbers of low birth weight infants are surviving, giving rise to a new epidemic of ROP. At present there is evidence of a variety of factors, in addition to oxygen therapy, that may contribute to ROP; thus the actual causes of the condition are still unknown.[8] The incidence of ROP in 1985 was reported to be at a level equal to the peak of the

RLF epidemic of the 1940s and 1950s,[6] with no indication of abatement in the near future. The current population of children with ROP are predominantly premature infants of very low birth weight (ie, 1,500 g). Although a newly approved therapeutic technique, cryotherapy, or freezing of portions of the retina, prevents severe visual damage in approximately one half of all treated eyes,[9] this treatment does not represent total remediation or prevention of visual impairment. Instead, the population of infants with ROP represents a group of children with partial sight at best, frequently accompanied by the constellation of potential cognitive, motoric, health-related, and neurological impairments observed in children of low and very low birth weight.[10–12]

While it is assumed that infant vision screening and early diagnosis can lead to intervention and treatment,[13] traditional pediatric examinations prior to discharge from the hospital include only pupillary light reflex, following of movement, and the clarity and health of the eye structure.[14] This type of examination allows detection of only the grossest impairments of the visual system. Palfrey et al reported that the mean age for identification of visual impairment (including blindness) by a physician was 54.9 months.[15] An earlier study by Jan et al, conducted in British Columbia on children born between 1944–1973 and categorized as blind, indicated that "parental suspicion [of a visual impairment] during the first year of life was almost the rule,"[16(p31)] implying a potentially significant discrepancy between functional and clinical detection of visual limitations. Furthermore, Gardner et al report that no states require visual testing of children under the age of 5 years.[17] Thus, unless educators and parents attend to visual behavior, including routine functional vision screening, the young child's vision deficit may not be identified until he or she enters school and visual learning demands increase significantly.

IMPACT OF VISUAL IMPAIRMENT ON DEVELOPMENT AND LEARNING

A review of the research literature reveals that there is only limited knowledge of how young children with visual disorders develop.[2,18–20] Furthermore, only two longitudinal studies of infants with vision loss have been reported, both addressing a very limited number of children.[21–22] While the dearth of research can be explained, in part, by limited population size and by the extreme heterogeneity of population characteristics, these research limitations have also impeded development of adequate screening and assessment measures as well as of systematic intervention techniques and effective models. That vision loss does indeed present a potentially severe barrier to the acquisition of cognitive and functional skills can be extrapolated from the literature that is available and from knowledge of the role of vision in learning and development.

Vision plays a major role in incidental learning; in extension of the learner beyond his or her own body; in the mediation of input from the other senses; and in the integration of a multitude of person, object, and environmental concepts such as color, size, shape, and position in space.[3] In infancy the role of vision is to motivate, guide, and verify the child's interaction with the environment. It serves to facilitate development of the ability to transfer information across the various sensory input systems so that the infant is able to obtain information from one sensory modality and apply it to another.[2,23] Vision is thus critical to all areas of development and learning. Moreover, the effective and efficient use of vision, including visual function and visual perception, is learned and follows a developmental progression. This learning is facilitated by the functioning of other sensory and neurological systems. Scholl reports that, at a minimum, "limited vision may yield imperfect sensations, which in turn yield imperfect perceptions that become vague impressions [that are] confusing to the educational process."[24(p67)]

The complexity and interdependence of sensory motor and cognitive processes are documented repeatedly in the developmental research literature. Impaired vision in infancy can result in a delay in the acquisition of early motor skills, because it deprives the child of motivation and accurate feedback as well as limits the use of imitation for learning.[24] In his extensive review of the literature on blindness and early childhood development, Warren reported multiple areas of potential developmental problems for children with visual limitations who do not receive early stimulation, stating that "sensory deprivation may be a particularly devastating condition, producing deficits not only in exploratory behavior and related learning and cognitive functions but also in the area of emotional development."[19(p17)]

Additionally, because of the role that the brain plays in vision, cognitive or neurological impairments can result in the dysfunctional use of vision, even by the child whose ocular structure appears to be intact. A child with a disabling condition is always vulnerable to impairments in the visual system. Children with unidentified or unaddressed vision limitations may be at risk of secondary handicaps, splintered skill attainment, or lags across the various developmental domains if they do not receive intervention such as stimulation and instruction, remediation, or compensation for the visual system deficits.

Many of the visual perception disorders associated with learning disabilities are similar to those seen in children with partial sight.[3] Given the interaction between the eye and the brain in the development and use of vision, undetected vision difficulties in early childhood (eg, muscle imbalance) may have a significant impact on the development of visual perception, leading to difficulties in reading and other academic and functional skills.[25–28] Rosenblith's research documented that infants with poor visual fixation and tracking skills demonstrate absence of visual memory at 8 months of age and poor performance on gross motor scales at 4 years of age.[29]

Indeed, the stability and importance of the healthy infant's visual–perceptual abilities have resulted in the use of visual fixation, tracking, and preference responses as indicators of later learning and developmental problems in childhood.[30]

ADDRESSING THE UNIQUE LEARNING NEEDS OF THE CHILD WITH A VISUAL IMPAIRMENT

The importance of development during the first 3 years of life for future competence has been well documented. The barriers to development imposed by a vision impairment are substantial, particularly in light of the role of vision in acquisition of a sensorimotor foundation.[31] The child with a vision loss is in need of intervention with two major foci: (1) ensuring that the limitations in vision do not interfere with development and learning; and (2) developing optimal functional vision. While these are not mutually exclusive goal areas, their implications for programming can be examined separately.

Children with visual impairments have unique needs that cross all developmental domains and curricular areas.[19,32] These needs encompass both learning the same things that all children need to know in ways different from those of the seeing child and developing a set of unique skills specific to the visual impairment. Because vision loss interferes with incidental learning and the use of visual modeling as a learning strategy, skills and concepts must be taught systematically and directly through the child's other senses. A common error in programming for the child with a vision loss is the assumption that hearing and touch correspond directly to vision in terms of the quality of information received by the child. Many programs substitute verbal descriptions and the use of models and other tactual materials for visual instruction, thus bypassing the strategies typical of the sensorimotor stage in favor of symbolization and other techniques more appropriate to the preoperational stage of development. The child with a visual impairment is at great risk of forming inadequate and inaccurate cognitive functions and concepts with which to interpret sounds, tactual information (eg, models), and so forth.

While the use of the child's intact senses is critical to the education process, instruction must ensure that the child (1) uses real objects as much as possible so that all sensory cues can be perceived; (2) has an opportunity to engage actively in all activities and experiences rather than, for example, just hearing them described, so that the child can form the constructs with which to interpret sensory input; (3) is provided with continuous motivation, guidance, and feedback throughout the learning process so that the child can ascertain the exact nature of environmental events and his or her relationship to those events; and (4) receives systematic, sequential instruction so that gaps in skill development and concept development do not occur. Children with visual impairments must be encouraged to move out into the environment and to interact with persons and objects in that environment. This encouragement ranges from tickling and cuddling the child to promote head raising while in the prone position, to physically guiding the child through crawling in order to reach a favorite food item or some other desired object. During typical interactions, such as when changing diapers, the child should be given the opportunity to discern the difference between a wet and dry diaper, how the diaper is removed or put onto his or her body, and so forth.

Attention to learning opportunities should also include feedback about what the child does. For example, if the child hits a toy accidentally and it causes movement or a change in that toy, attention should be directed to the change and repetition of the movement should be encouraged, with physical guidance. Information that is missed due to impaired observation should be provided in other ways. For example, the child's attention should be directed to each stage of the process of mashing up a banana for lunch, visually and/or tactually as appropriate. Getting juice out of the refrigerator or a clean shirt or diaper from a drawer should involve the child in some way, so as to ensure development of such functions as object permanence. As the child's skills develop, opportunities for practice and feedback must be provided and gaps in skills and concepts must be monitored by challenging the child to demonstrate an understanding of a concept actively, rather than simply to articulate it or imitate another's behavior directly.

During the early childhood years it is critical to ensure that the child develops the foundation required to benefit from instruction in the specialized concepts and skills needed for maximum learning throughout school and for independent functioning in adolescence and adulthood. In addition to the typical developmental, academic, and functional curricular areas in which the child must gain skill and knowledge, a child with a visual impairment must receive instruction in skill areas unique to his or her disability. These areas include (1) efficient and effective use of all senses, including sight; (2) orientation and mobility; (3) use of technological aids; (4) alternative forms of information access and output, including use of maps and models, braille, tape, large print, keyboarding, and other communication skills; (5) adaptive living skills; (6) adaptive prevocational and vocational skills; (7) social interaction skills; (8) adaptive recreation and leisure skills; and (9) self-advocacy and self-management skills.

As has already been discussed briefly, attention must also be paid to the young child's attainment of skills across the various domains that may otherwise be delayed or of poor quality. These include:

- Motor development: (1) prehension; (2) movement out into the environment; (3) head control and arm and upper body strength; (4) balance and gait; (5) position-in-space concepts.
- Language development: (1) vocabulary building, including use of adjectives and images; (2) expressions of feelings; (3) self-image and conceptual state-

ments; (4) sound localization and discrimination; (5) sound-symbol associations.

- Cognitive development: (1) concept development, including spatial relations; (2) causality; (3) object permanence; (4) classification; (5) conservation; (6) generalization; (7) symbolic representation.
- Self-help: (1) acquisition of all self-help skills; (2) independence in performance of skills; (3) evaluation of performance (eg, noting delays in putting on clothes, selecting clothes and dressing without prompting or other assistance, determining whether clothes match and are clean).
- Social development: (1) emotional expression and responses; (2) separation; (3) independence and self-direction; (4) self-esteem.
- Sensory development: (1) stimulation perception and discrimination; (2) directionality; (3) attention via all senses (visual, auditory, tactual, kinesthetic, gustatory, and olfactory).[32]

The role of the parent and the interventionist in ensuring that the child's learning is not significantly hampered by the access limitations imposed by a visual impairment can be conceptualized in part as that of a mediating agent, as defined by Feuerstein.[33] For the child with a visual impairment the interventionist must actively transform stimuli in the child's environment, and consequently the child's responses to those stimuli, so that the child is able to perceive, integrate, and act on the environment. To this end the parent, interventionists, and other mediators who interact with the child must not only facilitate the child's access to experiences and information and assist in the interpretation thereof, but must also do so through judicious modification of the environment and materials available to the child.

Attention to basic features of the environment such as lighting, glare, contrast, and the size of visual stimuli facilitates use of remaining vision. Controlling background or ambient noise and the volume, clarity, and rate of sound facilitates use of hearing. The organization and placement of objects in the environment, as well as tactual, auditory, and/or visual modifications to those objects, facilitate independent exploration and interaction. The use of consistent routes, scheduling, and other structures enables the child to anticipate and plan for events in the day and for their attendant instructional components.

The importance of effective and efficient use of the senses merits particular attention when developing goals and modifying the environment for the young child with a visual impairment. Two commonly held misconceptions about blindness are that it prevents all vision and that other senses become highly developed to compensate for the vision deficit. Sensory stimulation and sensory-efficiency training should be discrete and deliberate components of the child's curriculum and should also be infused into all other aspects of the child's day. While new concepts should not be taught through senses that are inefficient, every effort should be made to encourage more effective use of the senses during all activities. For example, bottles and other utensils used during feeding should be adapted to be visually exciting and accessible to the child in order to encourage focus, tracking, or other skills appropriate to the vision potential. Sensory stimulation should be meaningful and require active participation on the part of the child to ensure not only functional use of senses but also sensory integration and concept development through consistency of stimuli and direction of attention and interpretation. In an effort to render the environment stimulating and accessible, attention should be paid to gradually removing artificial sensory cues as the child's ability to access and act on sensory information increases.

IDENTIFYING THE YOUNG CHILD WITH A VISUAL IMPAIRMENT: A TEAM APPROACH

For the young child who is at risk for developmental delay or has a disabling condition, the initial contact with services is usually in the medical arena. Thus the family and early interventionist might assume that the child has been evaluated for visual function and that the lack of a diagnosis of visual impairment indicates intact sight. As the work of Palfrey et al[15] and Jan et al[16] implies, however, this may not always be the case, particularly in regard to those children with partial vision loss. Furthermore, because of the difficulty in determining the exact nature and degree of vision in a very young child, and the lack of mandates for vision screening, those children with severe vision loss who do not have severe ocular anomalies are also at risk for misidentification. Thus identification and implementation of appropriate intervention for this population of children is highly dependent on cooperation between the family and the medical and educational professions. Even when a medical diagnosis is provided, additional information about the child's functional vision is necessary to ensure that appropriate services will be provided. Briefly, the role of each primary team member in identifying the vision needs of the child is as follows:

- Family: The family is critical to providing information about how the child responds to visual stimuli; the nature of the stimuli to which the child responds; patterns of alertness, comfort, and discomfort throughout the day; preferred body positions; and other variables that affect how the child may use vision.
- Physician: The physician contributes information about the nature and prognosis of the eye condition, medical treatment, correction and/or management, documentation for service eligibility, interpretation of medical evaluations, and guidance with respect to health management and implications of the eye disorder.

- Educational specialist: Educational specialists address the child's functional use of vision. They can assess and document indications of vision and vision loss, assist the parents in identifying visual behaviors and describing the child's range of vision, justify referral for medical evaluation and provide data that can help the physician to identify vision characteristics and needs of the child, provide information about how best to work with the child during an examination, and assist the family and others in interpreting medical information.

It is critical to remember that any of the roles just listed can serve as the initial source for identification of the child with a vision loss. It should not be assumed that an in-depth ophthalmological examination has been done and that the absence of diagnosis means intact vision, even if the child has had extensive medical intervention. Thus any key person in the child's life may begin the process of identifying vision needs by documenting vision behaviors. A complete functional vision assessment should be carried out by an educator who specializes in visual impairments as part of any child's initial referral for early intervention services.[34]

The most important components of the total programming for young children with a visual impairment are the team of experts and the family. Beyond identification, a wide range of expertise can contribute significantly to the child's development.

Within the health care community, ophthalmologists and optometrists are critical to the medical management and correction or remediation of eye problems. These specialists, nurses, and other health care professionals can also provide valuable guidance in the maintenance of the eye and ocular aids, and in the identification of indicators of problems or changes in vision or health status.

Physical and occupational therapists provide direction for gross and fine motor development, particularly for attainment of prehension skills, posture and gait, head control, motor planning, and strength and stamina. If the child has an additional disability, these professionals' input is necessary to determine optimal positioning for sensory stimulation and use of the senses. Speech and language therapists can facilitate development of listening and other receptive language skills, vocabulary building, and qualitative attainment of language structures.

The early childhood education specialist and the educator in visual impairments, if not the same person, must work closely together to ensure that optimal development and learning occur and that necessary instructional and environmental adaptations, appropriate resources, equipment, and materials, and unique educational and curricular components are incorporated into the child's program.

Other vision specialists who should participate in the child's instructional program include the orientation and mobility specialist, who, in conjunction with the physical therapist, ensures that the child attains the necessary motor, cognitive, and conceptual skills for independent mobility. The independent living specialist, along with the occupational therapist, can ensure development of adequate self-help and daily living skills.

Social workers contribute assistance to the family and providers in accessing the health, educational, and financial resources that are necessary to the child, including financial assistance for procurement of needed equipment and services.

The most important resource for the young child with a visual impairment is, of course, the family. Because the family is the most consistent presence in the child's life, and thus the most appropriate mediator of the child's experiences, all other team members must perceive their roles as service to the family. Because a visual impairment merits ongoing services into adulthood, families should receive guidance and information regarding case management, advocacy, access to resources, and instruction and stimulation. Attention should be paid to meeting their informational, financial, emotional, and social needs so that they can incorporate their child into the family easily and provide the interaction and guidance necessary to learning and development. Most importantly, their goals, priorities, and choices should be solicited and addressed first when planning intervention for their child. Information should be provided to the family on eye conditions, prognosis, and implications of the vision loss; on resources such as parent groups, materials centers, and financial assistance; and on any other topics in which they have an interest. The wealth of specialists and materials that are potentially available to the child should be carefully coordinated so that parents are not supplanted or overwhelmed by visitors, technical information, and/or conflicting goals and priorities.

The need for systematic, consistent, and comprehensive experiences and instruction for the child dictates close cooperation, coordination, and communication among professionals. To this end, case management serves a key function in the child's life to facilitate service delivery, information brokerage, referral, resource access, and transitions to preschool and school. As the implementation of Public Law 99-457, the Right to Education for All Handicapped Children Act, Amendments of 1986, progresses, and services consequently become increasingly available and family-focused, the individual who assumes responsibility as the case manager for a young child with a vision loss must facilitate use of a system of diverse resources addressing multiple, diverse, and unique learning needs. This system should function to decrease rather than heighten the child's risk of splintered and inadequate skill attainment and development.

As has been discussed, children with visual impairment have unique learning needs requiring attainment of specialized skills for maximum independent functioning. Because a visual impairment is a "handicap of access," children with vision loss must also develop the same array of skills and concepts that are provided to all children through the educational process. Ensuring that the full scope of educational services is provided is thus fraught with a variety of problems and controversies. Problems in providing optimal services result from the array of specialized needs and the limited specific knowledge about how learning occurs in the absence of good vision. These problems are further compounded by the fact that the population of children with vision loss is limited in prevalence and highly variable in characteristics, and thus in learning needs. Consequently, many educational settings find it difficult to recruit and finance adequate staff and resources for a small number of vision-impaired children, despite what Public Law 94-142 may mandate. Those systems that do attempt to provide the full array of specialists often encounter difficulty because of the acute shortage of teachers and of orientation and mobility specialists. Teachers who have been trained in both visual impairment and early childhood are especially rare.

The low prevalence, personnel shortages, population variability, and wide range of educational needs further complicate identification of optimal settings and programs. There are many administrative, social, and skill-development benefits to both integrated and specialized settings for this population, resulting in controversy about optimal service models. Often the full scope of resources is available only in a setting where larger numbers of children can be brought to- r̃ethɲɾ ɑ̃ı̃ ḥ ɑ̃ɣ ɑ̃ ı̃ ɯ̃ḥ ıṇ̃ı̃ɑ̃ɩ ɯ̃ ḥ ̃ɑ̃ɩ̃ɩ̃ ɯ̃ı̃ɩ̃ɑ̃ɯ̃ɯ̃ɯ̃ **prɣɯɣḥɑ̃ɑ̃ɩ,** ḥ̃ɯ̃ɩ̃ɩ̃ɩ̃ı̃ı̃ı̃ḥ ̃ı̃ɯ̃ ı̃ ɯ̃ɩ̃ı̃ ̃ gated model also derives from the myriad of specialized skills that children with vision loss must develop beyond those required by all children. Many parents and educators believe that a more homogeneous setting allows more time and attention to be devoted to developing specialized skills. Conversely, while children with vision loss do need specialized instruction, they also require the full range of generic educational services, and they benefit greatly, both immediately and in the long run, from the opportunity to interact with nondisabled peers and to function in the integrated environment for which all facets of their education are preparing them. Thus, because of personnel shortages, low prevalence, and limited resources, educational placement decisions often require a weighing of specialized versus generic needs and of resource availability, resulting in a compromise of optimal educational programming. Until more is known about the nature of learning in children with visual impairments, and until all settings are able to provide the full range of specialized resources required by children with vision loss, the controversy and compromises will continue.

The implications of this dilemma are particularly relevant to providing early childhood services, in two ways:

1. Those same conditions that affect services and placement decisions for school-age children also affect early childhood services (ie, availability of trained personnel to meet specialized needs, time and opportunity to learn specialized skills, resource availability for a very small segment of the early childhood population). Thus providers must make decisions about how to design and staff services to ensure that the needs of the young child with vision loss are adequately met.

2. Early childhood services play a particularly critical role in laying an adequate foundation so that the extent of special needs will be minimal by the time the child reaches school age, thus enabling the child to benefit from the full range of typical as well as special education services offered.

Effective intervention during early childhood can minimize the developmental gaps and lags that often increase the child's needs for specialized services and reduce the child's ability to interact with and benefit from the kind of integrated setting that is available in many areas.

• • •

The young child with a visual impairment presents a unique set of needs. The risk of misidentification is great, particularly for the very young child and the child with multiple disabilities, and it dictates close attention to behavioral characteristics and close cooperation among the family, the medical community, the early childhood educator, and the special educator in the area of visual impairments.

Young children with visual impairments are at high risk for secondary handicaps, gaps in skill and concept development, splintered skill attainment, and poor developmental progression. Yet, because visual impairment is a handicap of access, most of the difficulties experienced by the vision-impaired child can be prevented or minimized through careful, systematic intervention from a coordinated resource and expertise pool and through specialized instruction in areas specific to the impairment. Interventions should include mediation of typical experiences and adaptations of the environment and objects in that environment to ensure that learning occurs.

The importance of providing consistent and comprehensive learning opportunities, as well as the diversity of child and family needs and of the resources available to meet those needs, demands close cooperation by everyone involved with the child and systematic case management across time. (Some resources are listed in the Appendix to this article.) Early intervention is critical to prevent developmental delay. Vision is frequently referred to as the unifying sense, the sense through which most learning takes place for individuals with intact sight. Loss of vision, although potentially devastating, need not inevitably result in dysfunction if adequate intervention is made available.

REFERENCES

1. Hill EW, Smith BA, Dodson-Burk B, et al: Orientation and mobility for preschool visually impaired children, in Tuttleton D (ed): *Yearbook of the Association for Education and Rehabilitation of the Blind and Visually Impaired: 1986.* Washington, DC, Association for Education and Rehabilitation of the Blind and Visually Impaired, 1987, pp 8–22.

2. Ferrell KA: Infancy and early childhood, in Scholl G (ed): *Foundations of Education for Blind and Visually Handicapped Children and Youth: Theory and Practice.* New York, American Foundation for the Blind, 1986, pp 119–137.

3. Barraga N: Sensory perceptual development, in Scholl G (ed): *Foundations of Education for Blind and Visually Handicapped Children and Youth: Theory and Practice.* New York, American Foundation for the Blind, 1986, pp 83–99.

4. Phelps DL: Retinopathy of prematurity: An estimate of visual loss in the United States, 1979. *Pediatrics* 1981;67:924–925.

5. Peyman G, Schulman J: *Intravitreal Surgery: Principles and Practice.* East Norwalk, Conn, Appleton & Lange, 1986.

6. George DS, Stephen S, Fellows RR, et al: The latest on retinopathy of prematurity. *J Maternal Child Nurs* 1988;13:254–258.

7. Terry TL: Extreme prematurity and fibroblastic overgrowth of persistent vascular sheath behind each crystalline lens. *Am J Ophthalmol* 1952;25:203–208.

8. Zierler S: Causes of retinopathy of prematurity: An epidemiologic perspective, in Flynn JT, Phelps DL (eds): *Retinopathy of Prematurity: Problem and Challenge.* New York, Alan R. Liss, 1988, pp 23–33.

9. Cryotherapy for Retinopathy of Prematurity Cooperative Group: Multicenter trial of cryotherapy for retinopathy of prematurity. *Arch Ophthalmol* 1988;106:471–479.

10. Kushner BJ, Gloeckner E: Retrolental fibroplasia in full-term infants without exposure to supplemental oxygen. *Am J Ophthalmol* 1985;97:148–153.

11. McCormick M: Contribution of the low birthweight infant to mortality and morbidity. Read before the Retinopathy of Prematurity Update 1985 Conference. National Children's Eye Care Foundation, Bethesda, Md, Nov 1985.

12. Teplin S: The blind infant, toddler and child. Read before the Retinopathy of Prematurity Update 1985 Conference. National Children's Eye Care Foundation, Bethesda, Md, Nov 1985.

13. Sherman J, Copper J: Advanced diagnostic procedures for evaluating type of visual status of the child. *J Am Optom Assoc* 1979;50:1139–1149.

14. Fulton R, Manning K, Dobson V: Infant vision testing by behavioral methods. *J Am Acad Ophthalmol* 1979;86:431–439.

15. Palfrey JS, Singer JD, Walker DK, et al: Early identification of children's special needs: A study of five metropolitan communities. *Pediatrics* 1987;111: 651–659.

16. Jan JE, Freeman RD, Scott EP: *Visual Impairment in Children and Adolescents.* New York, Grune & Stratton, 1977.

17. Gardner L, Morse A, Tulloch D, et al: Visual impairment among children from birth to age five. *Vis Impair Blind* 1986;80:535–537.

18. Vander Kolk CJ: *Assessment and Planning with the Visually Impaired.* Baltimore, University Park Press, 1981.

19. Warren D: *Blindness and Early Childhood Development*, ed 2. New York, American Foundation for the Blind, 1984.

20. Lewis V: How do blind children develop?, in Lewis V (ed): *Development and Handicap.* Oxford, Eng, Blackwell, 1987, pp 32–59.

21. Norris M, Spaulding PJ, Brodie FH: *Blindness in Children.* Chicago, University of Chicago Press, 1957.

22. Fraiberg S: *Insights from the Blind: Comparative Studies of Blind and Sighted Infants.* New York, Basic Books, 1977.

23. Rose SA: Lags in cognitive competence of prematurely born infants, in Friedman SL, Sigman M (eds): *Preterm Birth and Psychological Development.* New York, Academic Press, 1981, pp 255–269.

24. Scholl G: Growth and development, in Scholl G (ed): *Foundations of Education for Blind and Visually Handicapped Children and Youth: Theory and Practice.* New York, American Foundation for the Blind, 1986, pp 65–84.

25. Glass A, Holyoak K, Santa J: *Cognition.* Reading, Mass, Addison-Wesley, 1979.

26. Goldstein E: *Sensation and Perception.* Belmont, Calif, Wadsworth, 1980.

27. Wyburn C, Pickford R, Hirst R: *Human Senses and Perception.* Toronto, University of Toronto Press, 1984.

28. Lerner J: *Learning Disabilities: Theories, Diagnosis, and Teaching Strategies.* Boston, Houghton Mifflin, 1985.

29. Rosenblith JF: Relations between neonatal behaviors and those at eight months. *Dev Psychol* 1974;10:779–792.

30. Miranda SB, Hack M: The predictive value of neonatal visual-perceptive behaviors, in Field TM, et al (eds): *Infants Born at Risk: Behavior and Development.* New York, Medical and Scientific Books, 1979.

31. Piaget J, Inhelder B: *The Psychology of the Child.* New York, Basic Books, 1969.

32. DuBose RF: Working with sensorily impaired children, Part I: Visual impairments, in Garwood SG, et al (eds): *Educating Young Handicapped Children.* Rockville, Md, Aspen Publishers, 1979, pp 323–359.

33. Feuerstein R: *Instrumental Enrichment.* Baltimore, University Park Press, 1979.

34. Zambone A, Allman C: Accessing services: State procedures for identifying and determining eligibility of young children with visual impairments. *Top Early Child Spec Educ* 1988;8(3):75–85.

Appendix

National resource agencies

American Foundation for the Blind
15 West 16th Street
New York, New York 10011
1-800-232-5463 (1-800-AFBLIND)

Provides direct and technical assistance services to children and adults with visual impairments, their families, and professionals. Provides information and referral services. Operates the MC Migel Memorial Library, a reference library on blindness and visual impairments, and maintains the Helen Keller Archives, the major national archives on blindness. Publishes books, monographs, leaflets, and periodicals in print, cassette, and braille forms. Initiates and stimulates research to determine the most effective methods for serving individuals with visual impairment. Provides professional consultation to governmental and voluntary agencies. Conducts agency and community surveys to assist in the expansion and improvement of specialized services. Conducts institutes, workshops, and training courses for parents and professional personnel. Provides legislative consultation. Maintains a job index of employment positions held by persons with visual impairments. Maintains a technology database of users of technological aids across the country, and links users with potential consumers of technology (eg, voice output computers). Records and manufactures talking books. Develops, manufactures, and sells special aids and appliances. Sponsors public education program.

American Printing House for the Blind
1839 Frankfort Avenue
Louisville, Kentucky 40206
(502) 895-2405

National organization for the production of literature and the manufacture of educational materials for children with visual and multiple impairments.

Receives an annual appropriation from Congress to provide textbooks and educational materials for all students attending public school programs, including those in early childhood programs. Maintains a registry of children with visual impairments in the United States.

Hadley School for the Blind
700 Elm Street
Winnetka, Illinois 60093
(312) 466-8111

Provides academic and vocational education through free correspondence courses from 5th grade through postschool. Provides free correspondence course to parents of young children with visual impairments, as well as courses in microcomputers and sensory aids.

Howe Press, Perkins School for the Blind
175 North Beacon Street
Watertown, Massachusetts 02172
(617) 924-3434

Manufactures and sells the Perkins Brailler (manual and electric), standard or jumbo braille cells, the Perkins "Videoscope" closed circuit television, slates, styli, mathematical aids, games, braillevision books for children, maps, heavy- and light-grade braille paper, and other materials and equipment related to reading and writing.

National Association for Parents of the Visually Impaired
PO Box 562
Camden, New York 13316
1-800-562-6265

National association with local affiliate parent groups across the country for parents of children with visual and multiple disabilities. Publishes parent resource materials and a parent newsletter. Sponsors a national conference for parents every other year and regional conferences. Assists parents and professionals in identifying resources and accessing services. Engages in federal, state, and local advocacy on behalf of families and children with visual impairments.

National Library Service for the Blind and Physically Handicapped
The Library of Congress
1291 Taylor Street, NW
Washington, DC 20542
(202) 287-5100

Through regional libraries across the country (see local telephone directory)
distributes free reading material to anyone who cannot utilize ordinary printed
materials because of a disability. Materials are provided in the formats of talking
books, cassette tapes or records (playback equipment provided), and braille.
Conducts national correspondence courses to train sighted persons as braille
transcribers.

Recordings for the Blind, Inc
20 Roszel Road
Princeton, New Jersey 08540
(909) 472-0606

Lends taped educational textbooks at no charge to students and professionals
with visual or physical disabilities.

Effects of NICU intervention on preterm infants: Implications for movement research

Carolyn B. Heriza, EdD, PT
Vice Chairman and Associate
    Professor
Department of Physical Therapy
School of Allied Health Professions
St Louis University Medical Center
St Louis, Missouri

**LTC Jane K. Sweeney, PhD, PT,
    PCS**
Chief, Clinical Investigation &
    Research for Army Medical
    Specialist Corps
Department of Clinical Investigation
Walter Reed Army Medical Center
Washington, DC

THE IMPLICATIONS for practitioners of developmental intervention for preterm infants in a neonatal intensive care unit (NICU) were discussed previously by Heriza and Sweeney.[1] In that article, clinical studies[2-21] that focused on movement parameters and behavioral state were analyzed with respect to sample size, frequency and duration of intervention, specific characteristics of the intervention program, and outcome of intervention. Although the studies varied with respect to rationale, procedures, study population, and measures of effects of intervention, NICU intervention was found to enhance the development of preterm infants when both caregiver and infant were active participants. Moreover, preterm infants exposed to NICU intervention in addition to a home-based program had a better developmental outcome than those in only one or the other type of program.

In this article, the clinical studies referred to above[2-21] are analyzed with respect to research design and instrumentation. The specific parameters of the studies and the terms used in this discussion are outlined in the Appendices. The studies are grouped in the following categories: infant intervention studies,[2-14] mother–infant intervention studies,[15-18] and mother training studies.[19-21] Infant intervention studies are sequenced according to unimodal and multimodal sensory stimulation and date of publication; mother–infant and mother training studies are sequenced by date of publication. The implications for future research into infant movement are discussed.

RESEARCH DESIGNS

All reviewed studies used two types of subjects: experimental groups receiving therapeutic intervention and control groups not receiving intervention. Two recent studies[19-21] used full-term infants as comparison groups.

Individual studies may be classified as preexperimental, quasiexperimental, or true experimental.[22] The preexperimental studies reviewed in this article included the posttest only, nonequivalent control group design in which infants who re-

Inf Young Children 1990; 2(4): 29–41

ceived the intervention were compared with those who had not experienced the treatment, for the purpose of establishing the effect of the treatment. Either the infants were clearly assigned to groups, or no statement was provided on group assignment. A major flaw of the preexperimental design is its inability to determine if the groups were equivalent before intervention. If the groups differed on the outcome measure, this difference could have been a result of the selection of the infant groups. The quasiexperimental studies included a pretest, posttest; nonequivalent control group designs; or time-series designs in which either the groups were assigned to intervention or control conditions or no statement was made as to infant inclusion. The true experimental studies included traditional pretest, posttest; control group designs or posttest only; and control group designs or time-series designs in which infants were randomly assigned to groups. Recognition was given to measurement of the dependent variable by an examiner blind to group status.

Five of the reviewed studies were preexperimental designs[2,3,9,15,18]; six were quasiexperimental designs[4,6,7,11,13,14] of which two were time-series[4,14] designs. Nine were true experimental designs, including five posttest only, control group designs[8,10,12,16,17]; three were pretest, posttest; control group designs,[19-21] and one was a time-series design.[5]

In general, designs associated with "weak" experimental control produced greater treatment effects, whereas designs associated with more rigorous control produced smaller effects. This was particularly true when the outcomes of intervention were measured shortly after the treatment. When results were measured more than 6 months after the end of treatment, however, significant effects were derived from studies with rigorous designs.

Ottenbacher et al,[23] using metaanalytic procedures to measure the effectiveness of tactile stimulation in early intervention studies, also noted that the greatest effect of the intervention was recorded more than 6 months after the end of intervention. This "sleeper" effect was hypothesized to be related to the nature of the outcome measures used and the ability of these measures to discriminate performance in infants and young children. Another possible explanation is that infants receiving intervention may be more responsive to the environment, which would enhance the dynamic interaction between caregiver and infant resulting in greater developmental gains at later ages.

Future research

Design variables, which determine the effectiveness of treatment, are important factors to consider in the interpretation of the results of early intervention studies. When intervention research is planned, random assignment to groups should be considered to ensure that the groups are equal at the beginning of the treatment. If random assignment is not included in efficacy studies, the results of the studies will be difficult to interpret at best and biased at worst. Blind observation procedures should be incorporated to obviate the possibility of differential bias in the outcome measure. NICU intervention studies should continue for 6 months after discharge from NICU to account for an apparent latency effect in treatment outcomes.

None of the reviewed studies used single-subject designs, but they may be useful when heterogeneous groups of infants are being considered for study.[24] Results in group studies are evaluated in terms of the mean outcome of the treated groups versus the control group. Beneficial or nonbeneficial effects in a group of infants do not eliminate the possible harmful or beneficial effects to a single infant, which may be lost in the group data. Single-subject designs provide accountability for the efficacy of treatment outcomes[24,25] and ongoing immediate feedback for clinical decisions on the appropriateness of a treatment for an individual infant subject[24,26] versus the same "packaged" treatment for all infants. In addition, the study of the individuality among infants will increase understanding of the process of change as reflected by the dynamic interaction of the infant and caretaker in the environment.[27-29]

INSTRUMENTATION

Developmental and behavioral tests

The nature of the outcome measure and the capability of the test to discriminate age-appropriate movement parameters are instrumentation variables that must be addressed in the interpretation of research results and the planning of early intervention studies. Outcome measures used for neonates in the reviewed studies included: the Graham-Rosenblith Behavioral Test for Infants[30]: three studies[2,3,9]; the Dubowitz, Dubowitz, and Goldberg Clinical Assessment of Gestational Age[31]: two studies[6,8]; the Brazelton Neonatal Behavioral Assessment Scale (BNBAS)[32] (or an earlier version of the scale): 11 studies[7,8,11–13,15–17,19–21]; and the Assessment of Preterm Infant Behavior (APIB)[33]: one study.[14] Of these tests, only the Dubowitz and the APIB were developed to assess preterm infants. The Dubowitz gestational age assessment comprises two scales: a neurologic assessment scale that evaluates posture, muscle tension, and joint mobility, and a scale that assesses physical external characteristics. It does not evaluate spontaneous or elicited movement or behavioral state. The APIB, adapted from the BNBAS, was specifically designed to assess the behavioral organization of the preterm infant according to the theory of synactive development. Of the reviewed studies, only one[14] used this test as an outcome measure; the results favored the treated infants.

For older infants, the Bayley Scales of Infant Development[34] were used in all reviewed studies[3,7,10,13,14,16–18] with three exceptions[15,19,20] The Denver Developmental Screening Test[35] was used in Widmayer and Field's studies,[19,20] and the Cattell Infant Intelligence Scale[36] was the outcome measure used by Scarr-Salapatek and Williams.[15] Reports from recent research indicate that the normative data for the 1969 Bayley scales are now outdated and that additional and updated normative data are required.[37]

Alternative motor tests developed in the 1980s are the Peabody Developmental Motor Scales (PDMS)[38] and the Movement Assessment of Infants (MAI).[39] The PDMS is both a norm- and criterion-referenced developmental tool encompassing gross and fine motor skills from birth to 7 years. The PDMS has some advantages over the Bayley Scales in that normative data have recently been collected. In addition, the test has broader scoring criteria, and encompasses both gross and fine motor activities. However, Hinderer et al[40] suggested caution in using the PDMS as a dependent measure for research because of the high standard error of measurements (variability in test performance of individual infants). The MAI is a criterion-referenced test encompassing four areas: muscle tone (readiness of muscles to respond to gravity), primitive reflexes, automatic reactions, and volitional movement. Intended for clinical use with infants during the first 12 months, scores for the risk of cerebral palsy are available for 4-month-old[39] and, according to M. Swanson, PT (conversation, December 1989), for 8-month-old infants.

For early outcome measures, the Neurological Assessment of the Preterm and Full-Term Newborn Infant (NAPI)[41] and the Neonatal Neurobehavioral Examination (NNE)[42] may be appropriate. The NAPI addresses the infant's capabilities of habituation, movement, muscle tension, and neurobehavioral responses. Similar to the NAPI, the NNE evaluates muscle tension and motor patterns, primitive reflexes, and behavioral responses. Unlike the NAPI, however, the NNE provides a numerical quotient, which represents the neurobehavioral status of the infant and assists in clinical decision making with respect to the identification of infants at risk for developmental problems, the selection of intervention strategies appropriate for the functional age of the infant, and referral of the infant at discharge for appropriate intervention services. Two studies addressed the frequency of movement. Using videotaped observations, Barnard and Bee[7] demonstrated that infants who received a rocking bed and a recorded heartbeat sound had significantly lower activity levels than control infants at 4, 8, and 12 days of age and at 34 weeks of gestation. Solkoff et al[10] used a stabilimeter to count the frequency of movements. Infants receiving tactile kinesthetic intervention were more active initially than control infants, but by 6 weeks, no differences were found in activity level. These inconsistent findings may be due to several possibilities: the type of instrumentation, the type of sensory modality, and the intensity, frequency, and length of treatment.

Of the studies addressing behavioral state regulation, 11 scored changes in state according to the criteria of the BNBAS or APIB; one[12] used Thoman's criteria, one[6] used criteria derived from other sources, and one[4] used independent criteria. Not all studies indicated whether the examiners were reliable in using the BNBAS or APIB to score behavioral state. Field et al[12] did not state whether examiners used Thoman's criteria reliably; testers in Barnard's[6] study had 97% agreement in classifying states. Interrater reliability for changes in state averaged 90% in the study by Korner et al.[4] Behavioral measures were used to quantify approach versus avoidance behavior,[5] self-regulatory versus stress behavior,[14] and infant motility, startles, smiles, clonic mouthing, and high-amplitude tremors.[4] All studies reported a range of interrater agreement between 81% and 100% on behavioral measures.

Videotape methods and analyses

Observational analysis,[43] especially the use of videotapes, holds promise as a means of identifying at-risk infants and determining the efficacy of treatment. In contrast to developmental tests that address motor milestones and, in some instances, the quality of movement, videotape analyses hold the potential for analyzing movement in its component parts with respect to the context in which the movement occurs. Hopkins and Prechtl,[44] using a qualitative approach to movements, successfully described movement in 12 infants from 3 to 18 weeks of age, with an emphasis on form as well as consequence and orientation. Description by form topographically analyzes movement, that is, the patterns of movement of limbs and body, including regularity, duration, and frequency. Description by consequences and orientation analyzes the effects of these movement patterns on the infant's physical and social environment. Hayley,[45] also using a systematic procedure of recording and coding spontaneous movement, videotaped 42 infants from 2 to 12 months of age in various positions: supine, prone, crawling, sitting, kneeling, and standing. In each position, four parameters of posture and movement were described: static position, intermediate position, transition, and mobility. The relative frequency and duration probability for each of the four parameters in the six positions were calculated. Results indicated that differences in the relative frequency and duration probability were found at different ages. When these data were compared to those of an infant with developmental delay, the systematic coding system differentiated the movement of a normal infant from that of an infant with motor delays.

Kinematic analysis

Kinematic analysis, a descriptive analysis of a movement pattern, has also been used to analyze infant movement. A variety of movements have been analyzed, including the kicking and stepping of preterm and full-term infants,[46-50] changes in motor coordination during the transition from prelocomotion to crawling,[51] and gait pattern changes from initial independent walking to walking during the second year of life.[52–55] This form of analysis has also been used to identify the characteristics of reaching in infants between 34 and 36 weeks of age[56] and in infants studied from 3 to 9 months,[57,58] as well as the relationships between speech events and arm movements.[59] Kinematic analysis is a sensitive measurement system that quantifies the quality of movement by capturing the dynamic quality of the movement; describing the movement according to the objective kinematic parameters of time, velocity, amplitude, and acceleration; and providing a permanent record of the movement.[60] Kinematic analysis may also be a sensitive instrument for the identification of neuromuscular dysfunction at early ages and holds promise as a tool for determining the effectiveness of early treatment. Although this form of analysis has been used primarily in laboratory and research settings, with advances in technology, these techniques will be affordable and practical in clinical settings. Kinematic analyses can easily be integrated into clinical environments because of the minimal time associated with attaching markers to skin or bony landmarks, the immediate retrieval of data, and the "instant replay" of the movement when videography is used in conjunction. The permanent visual records can be reviewed for identification of early movement dysfunction, compared against recorded movement patterns of the same infant or other infants, and used to determine the effectiveness of treatment interventions.

•   •   •

A wide variety of designs and instruments have been used to study the effects of NICU intervention for preterm infants. In future studies, investigators are advised to consider using quasiexperimental or true experimental designs rather than preexperimental designs, blind observation procedures to measure outcome, and randomization of infants. Because of sleeper effects, infants should be followed for 6 months after NICU intervention to determine maximum outcome from the intervention. The increased use of single-subject designs is encouraged to incorporate repeated measures through 6 months of age and to allow the modification of intervention contingent on the infant's responses. As the growing and developing infant interacts dynamically with the environment, the ecology of the nursery should be addressed as a major variable, to be controlled or manipulated, when designing research protocols in the NICU.

Wide variability in instrumentation and motor outcome measures exist with little or no replication of methods from previous studies. The search continues for discrete measures of movement outcome in high-risk neonates, and participation by physical and occupational therapists in neonatal movement research is critical. Videography, including kinematic analyses, holds promise for greater precision in measuring motor outcome than the use of motor milestones from developmental tests.

Additional research information can be received from Marcia Swanson, Child Development and Rehabilitation Center, WJ-10, University of Washington, Seattle, WA 98195.

REFERENCES

1. Heriza CB, Sweeney JK. Effects of NICU intervention on preterm infants: Part 1. Implications for neonatal practice. *Inf Young Children.* 1990;2(3):31–47.
2. Neal MV. Vestibular stimulation and development of the small premature infant. *Nurs Res Rep.* 1968;3:1–5.
3. Neal MV. Vestibular stimulation and development of the small premature infant. *Communicating Nurs Res.* 1977;8:291–303.
4. Korner AF, Ruppel EM, Rho JM. Effects of waterbeds on the sleep and motility of theophylline-treated preterm infants. *Pediatrics.* 1982;70:864–869.
5. Pelletier JM, Short MA, Nelson DL. Immediate effects of waterbed flotation on approach and avoidance behaviors of premature infants. *Phys Occupat Ther Pediatr.* 1985;5:81–92.
6. Barnard K. The effect of stimulation on the sleep behavior of the premature infant. *Communicating Nurs Res.* 1973;6:12–40.
7. Barnard KE, Bee HL. The impact of temporally patternal stimulation on the development of preterm infants. *Child Dev.* 1983;54:1156–1167.
8. Kramer LJ, Pierpoint ME. Rocking waterbeds and auditory stimuli to enhance growth of preterm infants. *J Pediatr.* 1976;88:297–299.
9. Katz V. Auditory stimulation and developmental behavior of the premature infant. *Nurs Res.* 1971;20:196–201.
10. Solkoff N, Yaffe S, Weintraub D, et al. Effects of handling on the subsequent development of premature infants. *Dev Psychol.* 1969;1:765–768.
11. Solkoff N, Matuszak D. Tactile stimulation and behavioral development among low birthweight infants. *Child Psychiatry Hum Dev.* 1975;6:33–37.
12. Field TM, Schanberg SM, Scafidi F, et al. Tactile-kinesthetic stimulation effects of preterm neonates. *Pediatrics.* 1986;77:654–658.
13. Lieb SA. Benfield G, Guidubaldi J. Effects of early intervention and stimulation of the preterm infant. *Pediatrics.* 1980;66:83–90.
14. Als H, Lawhon G, Brown E, et al. Individualized behavioral and environmental care for the very low birth weight preterm infant at risk for bronchopulmonary dysplasia: Neonatal intensive care unit and developmental outcome. *Pediatrics.* 1986;78:1123–1132.
15. Scarr-Salapatek S, Williams ML. The effects of early stimulation on low-birth-weight infants. *Child Dev.* 1973;44:94–101.
16. Powell LF. The effect of extra stimulation and maternal involvement on the development of low birth-weight infants and on maternal behavior. *Child Dev.* 1974;45:106–113.
17. Brown JV, LaRossa MM, Aylward GP, et al. Nursery based intervention with prematurely born babies and their mothers: Are there effects? *J Pediatr.* 1980;97:487–491.
18. Resnick MB, Eyler FD, Nelson RM, et al. Developmental intervention for low birth weight infants: Improved early developmental outcome. *Pediatrics.* 1987:80:68–74.

19. Widmayer SM, Field TM. Effects of Brazelton demonstrations on early interactions of preterm infants and their teenage mothers. *Inf Behav Dev.* 1980;3:79–89.

20. Widmayer SM, Field TM. Effects of Brazelton demonstration for mothers on the development of preterm infants. *Pediatrics.* 1981;67:711–714.

21. Nurcombe B, Howell DC, Rauh VA, et al. An intervention program for mothers of low birthweight infants: Preliminary results. *J Am Acad Child Psychiatry.* 1984;23:319–325.

22. Campbell DT, Stanley JC. *Experimental and Quasiexperimental Designs for Research.* Chicago: Rand McNally; 1963.

23. Ottenbacher K, Muller L, Brandt D, et al: The effectiveness of tactile stimulation as a form of early intervention: A quantitative evaluation. *Dev Behav Pediatrics.* 1987;8:68–76.

24. Ottenbacher K, York J. Strategies for evaluating clinical change: Implications for practice and research. *Am J Occupat Ther.* 1984;38:647–659.

25. Harris SR. Research techniques for the clinician. In: Connolly BH, Montgomery PC, eds. *Therapeutic Exercise in Developmental Disabilities.* Chattanooga, Tenn: Chattanooga Corporation; 1987.

26. Gonnella C. Single-subject experimental paradigm as a clinical decision tool. *Phys Ther.* 1989;69:601–609.

27. Fogel A, Thelen E. Development of early expressive and communicative action: Reinterpreting the evidence from a dynamic systems perspective. *Dev Psychol.* 1987;23:747–761.

28. Thelen E. Self-organization in developmental processes: Can systems approaches work? In: Gunnar M, Thelen E, eds. *Systems and Development: The Minnesota Symposium on Child Psychology.* Hillsdale, NJ: Erlbaum; 1989.

29. Thoman EB, Becker PT. Issues in assessment and prediction for the infant born at risk. In: Field TM, ed. *Infants Born at Risk: Behavior and Development.* New York: SP Medical and Scientific Books; 1979.

30. Rosenblith JF. The modified Graham behavior test for neonates: Test-retest reliability, normative data and hypotheses for future work. *Biologia Neonatorum.* 1961;3:174–192.

31. Dubowitz LMS, Dubowitz V, Goldberg C. Clinical assessment of gestational age in the newborn infant. *J Pediatr.* 1970;77:1–10.

32. Brazelton TB. *Neonatal Behavioral Assessment Scale.* 2nd ed. Philadelphia: Lippincott; 1984.

33. Als H, Lester BM, Tronick EC, et al. Towards a research instrument for the assessment of preterm infants' behavior (APIB). In: Fitzgerald HE, Lester BE, Yogman MW, eds. *Theory and Research in Behavioral Pediatrics*, vol 7. New York: Plenum; 1982.

34. Bayley N. *Bayley Scales of Infant Development.* New York: Psychological Corporation; 1969.

35. Frankenburg W, Dodds J. The Denver Developmental Screening Test. *J Pediatr.* 1967;71:171–191.

36. Cattell P. *Measurement of Intelligence of Infants and Young Children.* New York: Psychological Corporation; 1960.

37. Campbell SK, Siegel E, Parr CA. Evidence of the need to renorm the Bayley Scales of Infant Development on the performance of a population-based sample of 12-month-old infants. *Top Early Childhood Educ.* 1986;6:83–96.

38. Folio MR, Fewell RR. *Peabody Developmental Motor Scales and Activity Cards.* Allen, Tex: DLM Teaching Resources; 1983.

39. Chandler LS, Andrews MS, Swanson MW. *Movement Assessment of Infants: A Manual.* Rolling Bay, Wash: 1980.

40. Hinderer K, Richardson PK, Atwater SW. Clinical implications of the Peabody Developmental Motor Scales: A constructive review. *Phys Occupat Ther Pediatr.* 1989;9:81–106.

41. Dubowitz L, Dubowitz V. *Neurological Assessment of the Preterm and Full-Term Newborn Infant.* Philadelphia: Lippincott; 1981.

42. Morgan AM, Koch V, Lee V, et al. Neonatal neurobehavioral examination. A new instrument for quantitative analysis of neonatal neurological status. *Phys Ther.* 1988;68:1352–1358.

43. Sackett GP. *Observing Behavior: Vol II. Data Collection and Analysis Methods.* Baltimore: University Park Press; 1978.

44. Hopkins B, Prechtl HFR. A qualitative approach to the development of movements during early infancy. In: Prechtl HFR, ed. *Continuity of Neural Function from Prenatal to Postnatal Life.* Philadelphia: Lippincott; 1984.

45. Hayley SM. Assessment of motor performance in infants. In: Wiehelm IJ, ed. *Advances in Neonatal Special Care Division of Physical Therapy.* Chapel Hill, NC: University of North Carolina; 1985.

46. Heriza CB. Organization of leg movements in preterm infants. *Phys Ther.* 1988;68:1340–1346.

47. Heriza CB. Comparison of leg movements in preterm infants at term with healthy full-term infants. *Phys Ther.* 1988;68:1687–1693.

48. Thelen E, Bradshaw G, Wara JA. Spontaneous kicking in month-old infants: Manifestations of a human central locomotor program. *Behav Neur Biol.* 1981;32:45–53.

49. Thelen E, Fisher DM. Newborn stepping: An explanation for a "disappearing reflex." *Dev Psychol.* 1982;18:760–775.

50. Thelen E, Fisher DM. The organization of spontaneous leg movements in newborn infants. *J Motor Behav.* 1983;15:353–377.

51. Benson JB, Welch L, Campos JJ, et al. The development of crawling in infancy. Paper presented at the Eighth Biennial Meeting of the International Society for the Study of Behavioral Development, Tours, France, July 6–10, 1985.

52. Clark JE, Phillips SJ. The organization of upright locomotion. Paper presented at the Biennial Meeting of the Society for Research in Child Development, Toronto, Ontario, Canada, April 25–28, 1985.

53. Forssberg H. Ontogency of human locomotor control: I. Infant stepping supported locomotion, and transition to independent locomotion. *Exp Brain Rel.* 1985;57:480–473.

54. Thelen E, Cooke DW. The relationship between newborn stepping and later locomotion: A new interpretation. *Dev Med Child Neurol.* 1987;29:380–393.

55. Sutherland DH, Olshen R, Cooper L, et al. The development of mature gait. *J Bone Joint Surg (Am).* 1980;62:336–353.

56. Von Hofsten C. Catching skills in infancy. *J Exp Psychol.* 1983:9:75–85.

57. Von Hofsten C, Lindhagen K. Observations of the development of reaching for moving objects. *J Exp Child Psychol.* 1979;28:158–173.

58. Fetters L, Todd J. Quantitative assessment of infants' reaching movements. *J Motor Behav.* 1987;19:147–166.

59. Dowd JM, Tronick EZ. Temporal coordination of arm movements in early infancy: Do infants move in synchrony with adult speech? *Child Dev.* 1986;57:762–776.

60. Hartis SR, Heriza CB. Measuring infant movement: Clinical and technological assessment techniques. *Phys Ther.* 1987;67:1877–1880.

Appendix A

Infant intervention studies

Author	Design	Subject selection	Subject assignment	Group variables (heterogeneous/ homogeneous)	Control/ comparison	Type of recording	Variables measured
					Research parameters		
Neal (1968)	Preexperimental (posttest only, nonequivalent control group design)	Sample of convenience from four hospitals	Not stated	Heterogeneous	Control group	Blind	Graham-Rosenblith Behavioral Test for infants at 36 weeks PCA.*
Neal (1977)	Preexperimental (posttest only, nonequivalent control group design)	Sample of convenience from four hospitals	Systematically assigned according to birth order	Heterogeneous	Four groups: A: Experimental group-imposed rocking B: Experimental group-self-actuated rocking C: Control group, fixed hammock D: Control group, no hammock	Blind	Graham-Rosenblith at 37 weeks PCA. BSID† at 6, 12, 18, and 30 months.

Research parameters

Author	Design	Subject selection	Subject assignment	Group variables (heterogeneous/ homogeneous)	Control/ comparison	Type of recording	Variables measured
Korner et al (1982)	Quasiexperimental (time-series design)	Sample of convenience	Not stated	Heterogeneous	Control group	Not blind	Visual observations of quality of movement on 3rd and 4th days of environmental and control conditions for 100 minutes after feeding.
Pelletier, Short, and Nelson (1985)	Experimental (time-series design)	Sample of convenience	Randomly assigned	Heterogeneous	Control on standard mattress	Direct behavior observation (10-second epochs)	Hand-to-mouth, facial grimace, startle, trunk arch, finger splay, arm salute.
Barnard (1973)	Quasiexperimental (pretest; posttest; nonequivalent control group design)	Sample of convenience	Not stated	Heterogeneous	Control group	Not stated	Dubowitz, Dubowitz and Goldberg Clinical Assessment of Gestational Age weekly through 35 weeks PCA. Behavioral rating of activity grouped into six states.

Research parameters

Author	Design	Subject selection	Subject assignment	Group variables (heterogeneous/ homogeneous)	Control/ comparison	Type of recording	Variables measured
Barnard and Bee (1983)	Quasiexperimental (pretest, posttest; nonequivalent control group design)	Sample of convenience	Assigned	Heterogeneous	Control group	Blind	BNBAS‡ at 34 weeks of gestation prior to discharge and 1 month after discharge. Videotape recordings every 24 hrs on days 1, 4, 8, 12; 34 weeks of gestation open crib. BSID at 8 and 24 months postnatal age.
Kramer and Pierpoint (1976)	Experimental (posttest only, control group design)	Not stated	Randomly assigned	Heterogeneous	Control group	Blind	Neurologic scale of Dubowitz, Dubowitz, and Goldberg; clinical assessment of gestational age (weekly). BNBAS weekly.
Katz (1971)	Preexperimental (posttest only, nonequivalent control group design)	Random from four hospitals	Systematically assigned according to birth order	Heterogeneous	Control group	Blind	Graham-Rosenblith scales at 36 weeks PCA.

Research parameters

Author	Design	Subject selection	Subject assignment	Group variables (heterogeneous/ homogeneous)	Control/ comparison	Type of recording	Variables measured
Solkoff et al (1969)	Experimental (posttest only, control group design)	Sample of convenience	Randomly assigned	Heterogeneous	Control group	Blind	Activity level by stabilimeter. BSID at 8 months PCA.
Solkoff and Matruszak (1975)	Quasiexperimental (pretest, posttest; nonequivalent control group design)	Sample of convenience	Not stated	Heterogeneous	Control group	Blind	BNBAS at days 14 and 24 of life.
Field et al (1986)	Experimental (posttest only, control group design)	Sample of convenience	Randomly assigned	Heterogeneous	Control group	Blind	BNBAS on day 12 (end of treatment period). Behavioral observation of sleep/ wake behaviors (Thoman's criteria) and presence of body movements on day 12.
Lieb, Benfield, and Guidubaldi (1980)	Quasiexperimental (pretest, posttest; nonequivalent control group design)	Sample of convenience	Systematically assigned: Group 1— control Group 2— experimental	Heterogeneous	Control group	Not stated Not blind	BNBAS prior to treatment and at discharge. BSID at 6 months corrected age.

Research parameters

Author	Design	Subject selection	Subject assignment	Group variables (heterogeneous/ homogeneous)	Control/ comparison	Type of recording	Variables measured
Als et al (1986)	Quasiexperimental (time-series design)	Sample of convenience based on selected criteria	Systematically assigned: Group 1— control Group 2— experimental	Homogeneous, infants at risk for BPD[II]	Control group	Blind	Behavioral measures of stress v self-regulatory on days 10, 20, and 30 after birth and 36 and 40 weeks PCA. APIB[§] at 1 month corrected age. BSID at 3, 6, and 9 months corrected age.

* PCA = postconceptual age.
[†] BSID = Bayley Scales of Infant Development.
[‡] BNBAS = Brazelton Neonatal Behavioral Assessment Scale.
[§] APIB = Assessment of Preterm Infant Behavior.
[II] BPD = bronchopulmonary dysplasia.

Appendix B
Infant/mother intervention studies

Research parameters

Author	Design	Subject selection	Subject assignment	Group variables (heterogeneous/ homogeneous)	Control/ comparison	Type of recording	Variables measured
Scarr-Salapatek and Williams (1973)	Preexperimental (posttest only, nonequivalent control group design)	Sample of convenience, first 30 infants who met criteria	Systematically assigned alternately to experimental or control group	Homogeneous (black, low SES)	Control group	Not stated	Brazelton-Cambridge at 1 week and 4 weeks. Cattell Infant Intelligence Scale at 1 year
Powell (1974)	Experimental (posttest only, control group design)	Sample of convenience	Randomly assigned	Black singleton	Control group	Blind except for BSID behavioral scale	BSID* (motor, mental, behavioral) at 2, 4, and 6 months adjusted age. BNBAS† prior to discharge.
Brown et al (1980)	Experimental (posttest only, control group design)	Sample of convenience selected on infant and maternal characteristics	Random assignment to one of these three groups	Heterogeneous	Control group at discharge, not at 1 year	Not stated	BSID at 1 year.
Resnick et al (1987)	Preexperimental (posttest only, nonequivalent control group design)	Sample of convenience with stated criteria	Systematically assigned based on hospital number	Heterogeneous	Control group	Blind (evaluated by different team)	BSID at 1 and 2 years adjusted age.

* BSID = Bayley Scales of Infant Development.
† BNBAS = Brazelton Neonatal Behavioral Assessment Scale.

Appendix C

Mother training studies

Author	Design	Subject selection	Subject assignment	Group variables (heterogeneous/homogeneous)	Control/comparison	Type of recording	Variables measured
				Research parameters			
Widmayer and Field (1980, 1981)	Experimental (pretest, posttest; control group design)	Randomly selected from labor records	Preterm: randomly assigned to one of three groups	Homogeneous: black, low SES, teenage	Control group	Blind	BNBAS* at 1 month. DDST† at 4 months. BSID‡ at 12 months.
Nurcombe et al (1984)	Experimental (pretest, posttest; control group design)	Preterm: sample of convenience based on infant and mother criteria. Full-term: randomly selected	Random toss of coin	Heterogeneous	Control group	Blind / Blind	BNBAS before test. BSID at 6 months.

* BNBAS = Brazelton Neonatal Behavioral Assessment Scale.
† DDST = Denver Developmental Screening Test.
‡ BSID = Bayley Scales of Development.

Recent advances in developmental intervention for biologically vulnerable infants

Forrest C. Bennett, MD
Professor of Pediatrics
Child Development and Mental
  Retardation Center
University of Washington School of
  Medicine
Seattle, Washington

WITH THE ADVENT in the 1960s of neonatal intensive care technology for low birth weight, premature, and other biologically vulnerable and medically fragile infants, professionals and parents have shown an associated interest in the health and developmental outcomes of these infants. Accepted medical intervention strategies have become continually more complex and more aggressively utilized, resulting in dramatic reductions in neonatal mortality for the smallest and sickest newborns.[1-3] At the same time, concerns about the short- and long-term neurodevelopmental prognoses for graduates of neonatal intensive care have increased.

Longitudinal outcome investigations confirm a persistent prevalence (ie, 10%–25%) of major neurosensory disabilities such as cerebral palsy, mental retardation, and visual or hearing impairments in surviving very low birth weight (≤1,500g) infants.[4,5] In addition, it is becoming increasingly apparent that close to half of these survivors manifest some of the new morbidities of prematurity (eg, language, fine motor, perceptual, socioemotional, learning, or attention dysfunctions) during early childhood and into the school years.[4-7] These so-called minor neurodevelopmental disabilities are likely to be exacerbated by coexisting environmental and psychosocial disadvantages (eg, poverty, single parent, teenage parent, parental substance abuse). In these increasingly common, doubly vulnerable situations, prematurity is likely to be highly predictive of school developmental and behavioral problems.[8]

The past two decades have seen an increase in both the number of clinicians involved and the number of programs aimed at optimizing developmental recovery during and following neonatal hospitalization and at preventing or ameliorating associated neurodevelopmental morbidities. Professional support has extended to the home environment, where family and community provide much of the support for survivors of high-technology care. This article addresses the most prominent clinical challenges facing professionals in neonatal developmental care and critically examines the results of intervention research.

DEVELOPMENTAL INTERVENTIONS IN NEONATAL CARE

Original approaches

The focus and form of early, nursery-based developmental intervention programs have markedly changed over the past 20 years. Throughout the 1970s, neo-

Inf Young Children 1990; 3(1): 33–40

natal developmental intervention strategies focused on infant stimulation.[9] The two primary goals of these approaches were (1) to compensate for intrauterine experiences lost as a result of premature birth and (2) to correct for the presumed sensory deprivation associated with prolonged care in the disruptive neonatal intensive care unit (NICU) environment.[10] While a review of published efficacy investigations reveals great interstudy variability in terms of the specific developmental interventions (independent variables) used, practically all reporting centers in the 1970s employed early supplemental stimulation in one or more of four major sensory areas.[11] In fact, the majority of investigations are of multimodal (ie, combined) sensory manipulations in more than one circumscribed area. They are almost exclusively infant-focused, that is, based on "doing something" of a presumed stimulating nature to sick or recovering NICU residents. Nurses in the NICU have been the principal intervention agents in most reports. Other providers include physical therapists, occupational therapists, early childhood special educators, and infant developmental specialists.

The four major sensory modalities variously incorporated into these original NICU developmental intervention programs include (1) visual stimulation (eg, decoration of the surroundings, mobiles with brightly colored objects), (2) auditory stimulation (eg, singing, music boxes, recordings of the mother's voice or heart beat), (3) tactile stimulation (eg, nonnutritive sucking, flexing, massaging, handling, positioning), and (4) vestibular-kinesthetic stimulation (eg, rocking and using oscillating beds, including waterbeds). Countless different combinations of these infant-focused interventions have been described and analyzed (eg, massaging, handling, and rocking; use of a rocking bed and heart beat recording; visual decoration and body rubbing; and bright mobiles, massaging, rocking, singing, and music boxes, representing all four sensory modalities). The number of individual protocols is almost limitless, and intervention programs further vary in terms of their specificity (or lack thereof) within a given sensory area. For example, one program may use a variety of vestibular stimulations in differing degrees and sequences, while another may assess the effects of vestibular stimulation as specifically provided by a motorized hammock or, alternatively, by an oscillating waterbed. Such marked variability between individual intervention programs seriously impairs both the interpretation and generalizability of their outcomes.

As with the specific combinations of sensory stimulations, great variability also exists in the reported onset, frequency, and duration of interventions. The timing of initial developmental intervention may be immediately after birth, or some relatively arbitrary starting point such as 14 days of age, or a time when the infant is deemed physiologically stable. Likewise, even though most studies have provided an intervention program taking place at least several times daily, some stimulations were given only during feedings, some were prescribed every 15 minutes regardless of the infant's readiness or state of alertness, and others were contingent on the infant's own activity and responsiveness. In terms of duration, typical intervention endpoints have included term gestational age, attainment of normal birth weight, or nursery discharge. Furthermore, while most interventions focused exclusively on supplemental sensory stimulations during the infant's initial hospitalization, in recent years an increasing number of programs also provide intervention protocols for parents that continue after hospital discharge into the home.

Comparing efficacy studies involving NICU developmental interventions is further hampered by limited information about subject selection and sample characteristics. Many studies have exclusively involved families of low socioeconomic status with predominantly young, unmarried mothers. Unfortunately, most have also involved relatively healthy NICU residents; infants who may theoretically benefit the most from intervention, such as those of extremely low birth weight (≤1,000 g) and those experiencing numerous medical complications, are quite underrepresented in most published investigations. Thus, the bulk of experimental evidence has been accumulated from infants who, biologically and medically, are at relatively lower risk and home environmentally are at higher risk.

NICU intervention investigations have employed a wide variety of outcome measures (dependent variables). These can be grouped into three broad categories: developmental, medical, and parental. Developmental outcome measures have included performance on standardized neurodevelopmental and neurobehavioral evaluations, performance on specific cognitive-sensory tasks (eg, visual orienting, auditory responsivity, recognition memory), sleep/wake state organization, temperament characteristics such as activity level and irritability, and neuromotor criteria such as muscle tone and volitional movement. The medical outcome measures typically assessed are weight gain, head growth, oxygen requirements, frequency of apnea, frequency of emesis, and length of hospitalization. Parental outcome measures have included the frequency of parental visitation and evaluation of the quality of the parent–infant interaction. In sum, critical appraisal of the NICU developmental intervention studies of the 1970s involves a search for effects within a complex mixture of structural, methodologic, sampling, and outcome variation.[12]

Not surprisingly, the reported results of these original studies are as various as the methodologies employed, and the outcomes reveal great variability in terms of their exact nature, extent, significance, and duration. One or more positive developmental, medical, and parental outcomes are reported in almost every scientifically credible, infant-focused study published during the 1970s (ie, "anything works"). However, the benefits of one particular intervention protocol are often not replicated in other investigations, and, because of frequently contradictory results, only limited generalizations can be made from most of these individual, isolated outcomes. Even two major studies that used very similar multimodal stimulations in all four sensory areas reported conflicting results. Scarr-Salapatek and Williams[13] found significantly greater weight gain and superior performance in measures of neonatal behavior for experimental group infants, while Leib et al[14] reported no significant group differences in the identical outcome measures. The two studies did both report significantly higher scores on assessments of mental and motor development during the first year of life for experimental infants. But even this general agreement in findings must be cautiously interpreted because of its short-term nature and because of other studies showing essentially no infant performance differences.[15]

Current approaches

Because of the continued lack of consensus about the effectiveness of NICU interventions based solely on an infant stimulation model, there has been a clear shift in focus and orientation during the 1980s away from original remedial approaches and toward more developmental, family centered interventions emphasizing and facilitating parent–infant interactions.[16] This shift in focus has occurred, in part, because of a shift in philosophy; whereas the NICU setting was once regarded simply as a source of sensory deprivation, infant care professionals now focus on the frequent overstimulation and inappropriate pattern of interactions intrinsic to this environment. The more recent, parent-focused model attempts both to facilitate the biologically recovering infant's optimal social functioning and to directly train parents to recognize the important stress and stability signals of their sick infant. NICU interventions aimed at improving the parent–infant relationship have taken various forms. Interventions usually include a component of infant preparation and readiness for intimate contact and a component of parent instruction in initiating dialogue and responding appropriately to the fragile infant's communicative overtures. With this contemporary evolution to more parent-focused strategies, parents and other family members are, naturally, increasingly involved in the overall NICU developmental intervention plan.

As an additional impetus to avoid a purely stimulation approach, Gorski[17] and others[18] have carefully documented potentially adverse side effects of indiscriminate intervention. The link between repeated, intrusive handling of the physiologically fragile infant and such deleterious complications as hypoxia, acidosis, apnea, bradycardia, and vomiting has been demonstrated. Increasing numbers of detailed investigations into the typical life and ecology of the NICU emphasize both the instability of the sick infant's autonomic nervous system and the surprising ease of exacerbating this instability by continual and unpredictable disruptions of quiet sleep. For example, when the fragile infant becomes overloaded with stimuli, he or she may withdraw, become rigid, or demonstrate signs of autonomic nervous system dysfunction. As a result, the infant becomes unavailable to its environment, becoming unable to obtain information or give positive feedback and, in turn, causing the parents and other caregivers to feel less competent and effective. Thus, it is critical that fragile infants engage in interactions without experiencing great physiologic, motoric, and homeostatic regulatory costs.

Armed with this important information, contemporary NICU developmental intervention programs increasingly promote an infant protection approach, which minimizes unnecessary handling and times contacts to coincide with infant readiness. Als et al[19] have reported very encouraging results based on this type of highly individualized approach in a small group of very low birth weight infants with bronchopulmonary dysplasia (ie, chronic lung disease). Experimental group infants receiving individualized care had significantly briefer stays on the respirator, improved feeding behavior, better behavioral regulation, and higher mental and motor developmental scores in comparison to control infants receiving standard NICU care. Als and colleagues teach and train nurses in incorporating individualized nursing care plans into the daily routines of the intensive and intermediate care nurseries. The specific components of this environmental neonatology model include reduction of excessive environmental stimulations (eg, light, noise, traffic), minimal handling protocol, use of facilitative positioning, promotion of self-regulation and state control, timing of daily routines to match autonomic readiness, and parent support and behavioral observation training.

The most consistent finding of early 1980s studies that were partially or completely parent-focused involved the positive facilitation of parent–infant interactions. Almost all of these studies[20,21] reported at least some significant, objective enhancement of the mother–infant relationship, with only Brown et al[15] failing to detect any group differences in interactional quantity or quality. Several of these studies[20,21] also involved home-based interventions following hospital discharge. Some of the most sustained intervention effects were best demonstrated in programs that continued through the transition process and into the infant's home, with close and considerable parental involvement. Brown et al,[15] discussing their failure with a combined infant- and parent-focused approach to involve socially disadvantaged mothers with their hospitalized infants, enumerated impediments to maternal participation, including lack of transportation to and from the hospital, need to care for older children at home, inability to leave home because of cultural concerns of their own mothers, and crises of daily living (eg, inadequate or no housing, lack of financial support). These observations keep individual, limited NICU interventions in perspective and challenge investigators to develop innovative, comprehensive, coordinated approaches to the complex task of optimizing the developmental and behavioral outcome of low birth weight, premature infants.

DEVELOPMENTAL INTERVENTIONS FOLLOWING HOSPITAL DISCHARGE

Several intervention programs for biologically vulnerable infants and their families have addressed these complexities and attempted to provide comprehensive developmental and support services following discharge from the intensive care nursery. These contemporary family-focused models merit individual review.

Barrera et al[22] have described the results of a year-long home intervention with low birth weight, premature infants and their parents following nursery discharge. Study subjects were randomly assigned to one of three groups: (1) an infant-focused intervention group with the objective of stimulating the infant's developmental level of functioning, (2) a parent-focused intervention group with the objective of improving the quality of the interaction between parent and infant, and (3) a no-treatment control group. In addition, a full-term no-treatment second comparison group was used.

Primary outcomes included measures both of the infant (ie, Bayley Scales of Infant Development[23]) and of the home environment (ie, Caldwell HOME Inventory[24]). All infants were assessed at 4, 8, 12, and 16 months of age, corrected for prematurity.

The results suggested that although both intervention approaches were effective in modifying some aspects of the home environment and, to a lesser degree, in improving infants' cognitive development as measured by the Bayley mental scale, the parent–infant interaction approach seemed to have the greater impact. Two other important observations emerged from this well-controlled investigation: (1) both premature intervention groups consistently outperformed the premature control group after 4 months of age in terms of cognitive development, and (2) the full-term comparison group clearly outperformed all three premature groups at each evaluation age on both the Bayley mental and motor scales.

Resnick et al[25] reported similar results following a developmental intervention program that began while low birth weight, premature infants were still hospitalized in the intensive care nursery and that continued into the home for the first 2 years of life. This curriculum-based approach was primarily parent-focused and aimed to enhance the quality of the parent–child relationship. Control group infants received all the postnatal care and referrals customarily given in traditional care. Experimental group infants scored significantly higher than control group infants on the Bayley mental and motor scales at 12 and 24 months of corrected age. These investigators[26] have subsequently concluded that it appears to be more developmentally advantageous to work directly with parents, modeling interventions for them to use with their infants, than to work exclusively with infants.

Their work has led them to the opinion that parents should be integrated into the developmental intervention program from the very beginning in the NICU so that they can learn to respond to the infant's cues and provide appropriate stimulation.

More recently, Rauh et al[27] reported surprisingly significant long-term effects at 4 years of age following a relatively limited intervention program during the first three months following discharge from the intensive care nursery. Specifically, the intervention program consisted of 11 one-hour sessions involving a NICU nurse, infant, mother, and father (when available) and designed to acquaint the mother with qualities of her infant's functioning in different domains. The program aimed to facilitate maternal adjustment to the care of a low birth weight, premature infant, and, indirectly, to enhance the child's development. While significant experimental-control group cognitive differences were not found at 12 or 24 months of corrected age (using the Bayley mental scale), they subsequently emerged in favor of the intervention group at 36 and 48 months of age (McCarthy General Cognitive Index[28]). Such robust late effects certainly require replication in a larger cohort of biologically vulnerable infants in order to be confidently ascribed to such a brief early intervention.

With a similar rationale, investigators[29] at the University of Washington are currently conducting a demonstration project, the Transactional Family Systems Model (TFSM), for medically fragile infants following hospital discharge. The primary goal of the home-based TFSM is to foster positive interactions between parents and their low birth weight, premature, and medically fragile infants.

The investigators help parents to become sensitive to their recovering infant's behavioral cues. Program staff assist parents in interpreting their infant's behavior and responding in an appropriate, contingent manner. The four basic intervention steps are (1) educating the parents about the significance of their infant's unique "body language," (2) helping parents to tune in to their own interactional style and how that affects their infant, (3) helping parents, through guided practice and encouragement, to adapt their interactional styles as their infant develops, and (4) documenting for parents their infant's unique physiologic and developmental progress over time.

One of the intervention program's unique features is the use of videotape technology to sensitize parents to their own caregiving and interaction styles and to the behavioral responses and capabilities of their infant. While a formal evaluation of this intervention approach has yet to be completed, preliminary data suggest that TFSM can effectively and efficiently be applied as an independent intervention complementing existing home-based services for medically fragile infants.

Finally, the most comprehensive, intense, controlled investigation ever performed of the effectiveness of developmental interventions for biologically vulnerable infants and toddlers has recently been completed.[30] The Infant Health and Development Program is an eight-site (University of Arkansas, Albert Einstein

College of Medicine, Harvard University, University of Miami, University of Pennsylvania, University of Texas Southwestern, University of Washington, and Yale University) collaborative clinical trial of a combination of health, developmental, and family services designed to optimize the long-term outcomes of low birth weight, premature infants. The entire program was coordinated by the National Study Office at Stanford University.

The specific interventions emphasized a family support orientation and included regular home visitation by a family educator throughout the infant's first 3 years of life, attendance at a full-day child development center between ages 1 and 3, transportation to and from this center, bimonthly parent education group meetings, and periodic health and developmental follow-up care from hospital discharge through 3 years of age. The overall intervention curriculum was coordinated at the University of North Carolina's Frank Porter Graham Child Development Center and was adapted from this center's extensive intervention experience with environmentally vulnerable infants.

The primary analysis study group consisted of 985 low birth weight, premature infants across the eight sites. Approximately one third of study infants were randomized to the intervention group, receiving all of the enumerated services, and two thirds were randomized to the follow-up group, receiving the same periodic health and developmental follow-up protocol from hospital discharge through 3 years of age but none of the educational interventions. Additionally, the study design called for differential enrollment according to birth weight; that is, approximately two thirds of randomized infants were relatively lighter ($\leq$2,000 g) and one third were relatively heavier (2,001 to 2,500 g). Birth weight was distributed evenly between the two study groups. Other initial status characteristics for which balance was sought in the randomization included gender, maternal age, maternal education, and maternal race.

A total of 908 study subjects (92.2% of the original group) were comprehensively assessed in terms of cognitive, behavioral, and health outcomes at 36 months of age (corrected for prematurity) by evaluators unaware of the child's group assignment. Intervention group children performed significantly better on the Stanford-Binet Intelligence Scale[31] than follow-up group children. The effect of the intervention varied significantly with birth weight; the heavier intervention group scored an average of 13.2 intelligence quotient (IQ) points higher than the heavier follow-up group, while the lighter intervention group scored an average of 6.6 IQ points higher than the lighter follow-up group (both highly statistically significant intervention–follow-up group differences). Mothers of intervention group children reported significantly fewer behavior problems on the Achenbach Child Behavior Checklist[32] than mothers of follow-up group children. No significant group differences were found in growth parameters, scales of health status, or incidence of serious health conditions.

•   •   •

The Infant Health and Development Program and other developmental intervention programs following hospital discharge adequately demonstrate the useful-
ness of helping families to help their biologically vulnerable infants. Most successful programs have used a comprehensive combination of family support,
parent education, and child development approaches. While it is virtually impossible in most of these programs to specifically relate positive outcome effects to
individual components of the overall intervention plan, it seems highly probable
that, in fact, these broad, complex approaches are more likely to result in meaningful, persistent improvements than are narrow, simplistic approaches.

It is also probable that successful developmental intervention programs for this
population, like those for environmentally vulnerable infants, will be costly in
terms of both human resources and financial expenditures. Therefore, these efforts
should be directed to the target population most likely to benefit, that is, to those
doubly vulnerable infants at combined biologic and environmental risk. Simultaneously, programs that have demonstrated developmental effectiveness in the first
3 years of life must attempt to maintain their cohorts in order to critically evaluate
the preschool and school-age outcomes following the termination of early interventions.

REFERENCES

1. Hack M, Fanaroff AA, Merkatz IR. The low birth weight infant—Evolution of a changing outlook. *N Engl J Med.* 1979;301:1162–1165.

2. McCormick MC. The contribution of low birth weight to infant mortality and childhood morbidity. *N Engl J Med.* 1985;312:82–90.

3. Hack M, Fanaroff AA. Changes in the delivery room care of the extremely small infant (<750 g):
   Effects on morbidity and outcome. *N Engl J Med.* 1986;314:660–664.

4. Bennett FC. Neurodevelopmental outcome in low birth weight infants: The role of developmental
   intervention. In: Guthrie RD, ed. *Neonatal Intensive Care.* New York, NY: Churchill Livingstone;
   1988.

5. McCormick MC. Long-term follow-up of infants discharged from neonatal intensive care units.
   JAMA. 1989;261:24–31.

6. Dunn HG, Crichton J, Grunau R, et al. Neurological, psychological and educational sequelae of
   low birth weight. *Brain Dev.* 1980;2:57–67.

7. Blackman JA, Lindgren S, Hein H, Harper DC. Long-term surveillance of high risk children. *Am
   J Dis Child.* 1987;141:1293–1299.

8. Escalona SK. Babies at double hazard: Early development of infants at biologic and social risk.
   Pediatrics. 1982;70:670–675.

9. Meisels SJ, Jones SN, Stiefel GS. Neonatal intervention: Problem, purpose, and prospects. *Top
   Early Child Spec Educ.* 1983;3(1):1–13.

10. Gottfried AW, Wallace-Lande P, Sherman-Brown S. Physical and social environment of newborn
    infants in special care units. *Science.* 1981;214:637–675.

11. Field TM. Supplemental stimulation of preterm neonates. *Early Hum Dev.* 1980;4:301–314.

12. Bennett FC. The effectiveness of early intervention for infants at increased biological risk. In: Guralnick MJ, Bennett FC, eds. *The Effectiveness of Early Intervention for At-Risk and Handicapped Children.* Orlando, Fla: Academic Press; 1987.

13. Scarr-Salapatek S, Williams ML. The effects of early stimulation on low birth weight infants. *Child Dev.* 1973;44:94–101.

14. Leib SA, Benfield DG, Guidubaldi J. Effects of early intervention and stimulation on the preterm infant. *Pediatrics.* 1980;66:83–90.

15. Brown J, LaRossa M, Aylward G, Davis DJ, Rutherford PK, Bakeman R. Nursery-based intervention with prematurely born babies and their mothers: Are there effects? *J Pediatr.* 1980;97:487–491.

16. Ramey CT, Bryant DM, Sparling JJ, Wasik BH. A biosocial system perspective on environmental interventions for low birth weight infants. *Clin Obstet Gynecol.* 1984;27:672–692.

17. Gorski PA, Hole WT, Leonard CH, Martin JA. Direct computer recording of premature infants and nursery care: Distress following two interventions. *Pediatrics.* 1983;72:198–202.

18. Long JG, Philip AG, Lucey JF. Excessive handling as a cause of hypoxemia. *Pediatrics.* 1980;65:203–207.

19. Als H, Lawhon G, Brown E, et al. Individualized behavioral and environmental care for the very low birth weight preterm infant at high risk for bronchopulmonary dysplasia: Neonatal intensive care unit and developmental outcome. *Pediatrics.* 1986;78:1123–1132.

20. Bromwich RM, Parmelee AH. An intervention program for preterm infants. In: Field TM, ed. *Infants Born At Risk.* New York, NY: Spectrum Publications; 1979.

21. Field TM, Widmayer SM, Stinger S, Ignatoff E. Teenage, lower class, black mothers and their preterm infants: An intervention and developmental follow-up. *Child Dev.* 1980;51:426–436.

22. Barrera ME, Rosenbaum PL, Cunningham CE. Early home intervention with low birth weight infants and their parents. *Child Dev.* 1986;57:20–33.

23. Bayley N. *Manual for the Bayley Scales of Infant Development.* New York, NY: Psychological Corporation; 1969.

24. Caldwell BM, Bradley RH. *Home Observation for Measurement of the Environment.* Little Rock, Ark: University of Arkansas Press; 1979.

25. Resnick MB, Eyler FD, Nelson RM, Eitzman DV, Bucciarelli RL. Developmental intervention for low birth weight infants: Improved early developmental outcome. *Pediatrics.* 1987;80:68–74.

26. Resnick MB, Armstrong S, Carter RL. Developmental intervention program for high-risk premature infants: Effects on development and parent–infant interactions. *J Dev Behav Pediatr.* 1988;9:73–78.

27. Rauh VA, Achenbach TM, Nurcombe B, Howell CT, Teti DM. Minimizing adverse effects of low birth weight: Four-year results of an early intervention program. *Child Dev.* 1988;59:544–553.

28. McCarthy D. *Manual for the McCarthy Scales of Children's Abilities.* New York, NY: Psychological Corporation; 1972.

29. Hedlund R. *The Transactional Family System Program.* Unpublished mimeo. Seattle, Wash: Child Development and Mental Retardation Center, University of Washington; nd.

30. The Infant Health and Development Program. Enhancing the outcomes of low birthweight, premature infants: A multi-site randomized trial. *JAMA.* (June 13,1990).

31. Terman LM, Merrill MA. *Stanford-Binet Intelligence Scale. Manual for the Third Revision, Form L-M.* Boston, Mass: Houghton Mifflin; 1973.

32. McConaughy SH, Achenbach TM. *Practical Guide for the Child Behavior Checklist and Related Materials.* Burlington, Vt: University of Vermont, Department of Psychiatry; 1988.

Identifying and treating aggressive preschoolers

Sarah Landy, PhD
Beechgrove Children's Centre
Brockville, Ontario
Canada

Ray DeV. Peters, PhD
Queen's University
Kingston, Ontario
Canada

A MAJOR CHALLENGE currently facing society is that of finding successful treatment strategies for conduct-disordered, delinquent, and aggressive children, adolescents, and adults. Epidemiologic studies in a number of countries have found a prevalence rate of between 4% and 10%.[1-3] Of boys referred to children's mental health centers, it is estimated that 50% to 75% have a diagnosis of conduct disorder.[3,4] Aggressive behavior problems are a concern not only in terms of incidence but also in terms of continuity and prognosis. In 1979, Olweus[5] reported the stability of antisocial behavior through childhood and adolescence to be comparable in magnitude to that of intelligence. It is similarly estimated by other writers[6-9] that at least 50% of children identified as having aggressive conduct disorders will have serious problems in later life. Although the pathway from early conduct problems to later maladaptive adjustment is complex and remains to be clearly delineated, there are some longitudinal studies showing that children identified as hyperaggressive as preschoolers prove to be the most difficult to treat and their disorders the most intractable.[7,10-13]

Antisocial children contribute disproportionately as adults to the incidence of alcoholism, accidents, chronic unemployment, divorce, physical and psychiatric illness, and demand on welfare services. Overall, this mental health problem may cost society more financially and in emotional suffering than any other single disorder. There is no doubt that it is a source of great anguish to many individuals and their families and may pose a threat to the stability of our society.

IMPROVING PROGNOSIS WITH EARLY INTERVENTION

One reason for the high degree of continuity found in conduct disorders from childhood to adulthood has been the failure to find successful treatment strategies, particularly for children and families who are showing extreme dysfunction. Attempts at treatment for older children have been wide ranging, from individualized behavior management or cognitive treatment programs for the child to medication, family work, and community rehabilitation. Treatment strategies that have been most successful to date are those that target parent–child interactions (eg, parent management training or functional family therapy) or interpersonal, cognitive, problem-solving deficits within the child. Even these successes are limited to certain groups, and for a number of techniques there is little evidence to suggest

Inf Young Children 1990; 3(2): 24–38
© 1990 Aspen Publishers, Inc.

any positive behavioral change.[14] In general, treatment of the aggressive behavior-disordered child or adolescent works best with motivated, capable, middle-class families in which the problems are mild to moderate, rather than severe.[14]

Given the magnitude and pervasiveness of the problem of aggressive behavior disorders and the overall poor results of treatments geared toward the school-age child, two alternate approaches deserve attention. One approach involves the identification of at-risk young children before they manifest aggressive behaviors and the introduction of interventions designed to prevent the development of subsequent, disruptive behavior disorders. A second approach, to which this article is addressed, involves the identification and treatment of aggressive behaviors at earlier developmental levels, when they are less firmly established, and before correlated problems of peer rejection and poor school performance begin to sustain and compound them.

IDENTIFICATION AND SCREENING OF AGGRESSIVE PRESCHOOLERS

Because of the externalizing nature of many of their symptoms, aggressive preschoolers are readily identified by parents and day-care workers. Their behavior is characterized by unprovoked physical attacks on other children and adults, destruction of other children's property, frequent and intense temper tantrums, disrespect, noncompliance, and extreme impulsivity. These characteristics have been clearly described by researchers,[15-19] as well as in a number of case studies.[20-23]

As these writers point out, aggressive preschoolers have not developed strategies for dealing with frustration and anxiety without resorting to physical means and exhibiting affective disorganization. Acting out is usually not modulated through the use of language and rich sequences of pretend-play. These children seem fixated at an earlier, egocentric stage of development and are unable to differentiate their own needs from those of others and incapable of understanding or showing empathy for the feelings of other people. Similarly, aggressive preschoolers have not begun to internalize external standards or rules that can enable them to control aggressive behavior. Because these symptoms are so commanding of attention, the underlying chronic apprehension of the world, fragile self-esteem, anxiety, fearfulness, neediness, and sense of aloneness that may also characterize these children often go unnoticed.[16-18]

In addition to identification of these children at home and nursery school, a number of assessment tools are available that can be used to screen large numbers of children and to identify those with extreme aggression and other externalizing behaviors. Table 1 lists and describes a number of screening tools that have ad-

Table 1. Preschool screening instruments

Name of test	Age range	Time to administer	Purpose/ description comment	Ordering information
Test of Early Social and Emotional Development	3–8 y	10 min	Parent rating scale; recently normed; detects degree of behavioral difficulty	Pro: Ed, Inc. 5341 Industrial Oaks Blvd. Austin, TX 78735
Pre-school Behavior Rating Scale	3–6 y	10 min	Rated by preschool teacher in psychomotor, cognitive, and social areas; 20 items	Child Welfare League of America 67 Irving Place New York, NY 10003
Eyberg Child Behavior Inventory	2–12 y	10 min	Especially useful to measure child conduct problems and oppositional behavior; parent-rated scale	Sheila Eyberg, PhD Dept. of Clinical Psychology Box J165-JHMHC University of Florida Gainesville, FL 32610-0165
Kohn Problem Checklist	3–6 y	5 min	Teachers rate children on 49 problem behaviors	Martin Kohn William Alanson White Institute 20 West 74th Street New York, NY 10023
Behavioral Screening Questionnaire	3–5 y	10–20 min	60 questions asked in parent interview; to determine presence/absence and frequency/ severity of symptoms	N. Richman Dept. of Psychological Medicine Hospital for Sick Children Great Ormond Street London, WCIN 3JH, UK
Preschool Behavior Questionnaire	3–6 y	10 min	30-item teacher-rated scale of pervasiveness of behavioral problems	Lenore Behar 1821 Woodburn Road Durham, NC 27705

equate validity and reliability, are brief, and require no specialized expertise to administer.

These questionnaires can be used to identify children who are judged by parents or teachers to be displaying extreme aggression and noncompliance. Care is necessary to avoid labeling as hyperaggressive children who may be showing temporary symptoms in response to a crisis situation or a stage that they will overcome.

ASSESSMENT OF AGGRESSIVE PRESCHOOLERS AND THEIR FAMILIES

After the initial identification, more in-depth assessment will be necessary to ascertain the nature and character of the problems in the child, the family, and the environment surrounding the family, to understand those problems' unique influence and contribution, and, if necessary, to recommend treatment strategies. Assessments typically involve observations of the child and family in natural settings, such as home, nursery school, and the playroom. More in-depth testing should also be carried out by a number of different clinicians, such as physical therapists, nurses, psychologists, and other pediatric mental health specialists.

Table 2 lists assessment instruments that can be used to quantify and structure multidisciplinary assessments and to derive data on the most salient developmental characteristics of the child and the most important aspects of his or her interaction with the parents. Concurrent validity for these tests is well established, but in many cases, a lack of longitudinal data makes predictive validity hard to determine.

By the time preschoolers are identified as having excessively aggressive behavior, they are usually caught up in a cycle of acting out, which results in negative responses or excessive punishment by parents, a perception by the child of being rejected, and further acting out. This pattern frequently spreads to interactions with teachers and peers. It is as if the child continually confirms his view of himself and the world as "bad" and perpetuates that perception with expanding cycles of rejection (Fig 1).

Each case presents an enormous diagnostic challenge and dilemma of sorting out the relative contributions of organic and environmental factors within the cycle and the comparative role of relationship problems and cognitive deficits within the child. Areas that need to be assessed are

- the child's characteristics,
- parent–child interaction and relationship,
- the personality structure and marital relationship of the parents, and
- social and environmental factors.

The child's characteristics

Every preschooler referred for treatment of extreme aggression has failed to develop a number of critical capacities that are needed for increased control of acting out and mediation of anger through internal psychologic factors. The reasons for this developmental lag vary significantly, and each child has a unique blend of strengths and deficits.[16] Through observation and formalized testing, assessment procedures should identify the missing critical characteristics and the

Table 2. Assessment tools for hyperaggressive preschoolers

Name of test	Age range	Time to administer	Purpose/ description comment	Ordering information
Kohn Social Competence Scale	3–6 y	15 min or less	Teachers rate children on social competence in preschool setting; 73 items	Martin Kohn William Alanson White Instit. 20 West 74th Street New York, NY 10023
Pictoral Scale of Perceived Competence and Social Acceptance for Young Children	Pre-school– 2nd grade	10 min	Self-evaluation of perceived competence in cognitive and physical skills	Susan Harter Department of Psychol-ogy University of Denver 2040 S. York Street Denver, CO 80208
Lowe and Costello Symbolic Play Test	0–4 y	30 min	To measure level of *symbolic play*	N.F.E.R. Nelson Pub. Co. Ltd. 2 Jennings Bldg., Thames Ave. Windsor, Berks, SL4 1QS UK
California Child Q-Sort	3+ y	20–40 min	Gives measures of *ego-resiliency and ego-control* from battery of laboratory tasks; measure: self-control and adaptability	Consulting Psychologist Press 577 College Avenue Palo Alto, CA 94306
Child Behavior Checklist	2+ y	30–40 min	Records behavior problems and competencies of children	T.M. Achenbach University of Vermont 1 S. Prospect Street Burlington, VT 05401
Burks' Behavior Rating Scales: Preschool and Kindergarten	3–6 y	20–30 min	18 scales are measured; filled by parent (eg, anger control, impulse control, ego strength, aggres-siveness)	Western Psychological Serv. 12031 Wilshire Blvd. Los Angeles, CA 90025

continues

Table 2. continued

Name of test	Age range	Time to administer	Purpose/ description comment	Ordering information
Family Assessment Device	N/A	10 min	Gives a level of *family functioning*	Chedoke McMaster Hospital Chedoke Unit Box 2000, Station "A" Hamilton, ON L8N 3Z5 Canada Attn: Dr. Boyle or Dr. Offord
Home Observation for Measurement of Environment	Birth– 10 y	30 min	Measures home environment on 8 scales including stimulation, warmth and acceptance, variety; to assess the home and obtain an overall scale score	Center of Research University of Arkansas 33rd and University Little Rock, AR 72204 Attn: Bettye M. Caldwell or Robert H. Bradley
Procidana Perceived Social Support Questionnaire	N/A	10 min	Gives measures of perceived support from friends and family	Mary E. Procidana Department of Psychology Fordham University Bronx, NY 10458
Parenting Stress Index	N/A	20 min	Picks up risk for dysfunctional parenting	Pediatric Psychology Press 2915 Idlewood Drive Charlottesville, VA 22901
Family Resource Scale	Households with young children	5–10 min	Useful scale to measure parental health and wellbeing	Dr. C. Dunst Family, Infant & Preschool Western Carolina Center Morganton, NC 28655
Dyadic Parent– Child Interaction Coding System	2–10 y	15 min	Assess parenting skills and re- sponses to child's behaviors	Donald N. Bersoff 274 Sherman Avenue New Haven, CT 06511

continues

Table 2. continued

Name of test	Age range	Time to administer	Purpose/ description comment	Ordering information
Parent Behavior Rating Scale	N/A	15 min	Assesses parent's enjoyment, sensitivity, responsiveness with child	Dr. Gerald Mahoney Project Interact Dept. of Pediatrics Univ. of Connecticut Health 270 Farmington Ave., #164 Farmington, CT 06032
Q-Sort Measure of Attachment Assessment	1–4 y	20 min	100-item Q-set of affect, cognition, and behavior on attachment domain; parent sorts cards	Deane, K. and Waters, E. State University of N.Y. Stoney Brook, NY 11794
Positive Reinforcement Observation Schedule	Unrestricted		Amount of positive reinforcement	Dr. C. Dunst Family, Infant & Preschool Western Carolina Center Morganton, NC 28655
Empathy Task	3–8 y	10 min	Score reflects child's awareness of others' feelings	Helen Borke Psychology Department Carnegie-Mellon University Pittsburgh, PA 15213
Kansas Reflection-Impulsivity Scale for Preschoolers	3–5.5 y	10 min	Cognitive task requiring child to match figures in order to measure reflection/ impulsivity	CEMREL Inc. 3120 59th Street St. Louis, MO 63139
Non-verbal Measures of Children's Frustration	3.5–7 y	10–15 min	Gives scores on use of aggression, prosocial and avoidance choices	Fred W. Vondracek Beecher House Pennsylvania State University University Park, PA 16802

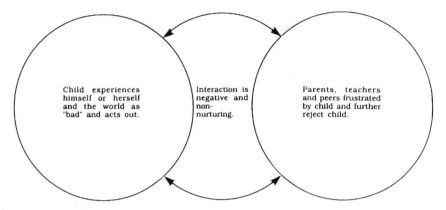

Fig 1. Cycle of rejection.

etiology of the child's developmental failures. Delays of development in these children may be due primarily to neurologic or physiologic problems[24-26] or to attachment disorders resulting from previous interactional difficulties. These problems may lead to difficulties in interacting with others, delays in symbolization (such as language and pretend-play), and failures in impulse control.[16] Children may exhibit only one of these factors or, in some cases, as many as three.

A number of researchers have found significant relationships between attachment insecurity and behavioral difficulties.[19,27,28] Children with attachment or relationship disorders may have experienced rejection by or losses of primary caregivers or various levels of insensitive parenting. As a consequence, they have a lack of trust and have failed to develop a positive mental representation or memory of earlier interactions that can sustain them in times of stress. For these children, it is as if an earlier sense of rage and deprivation continually demands expression in the present.[15] On the other hand, some children may show warmth and relatedness in interactions but have difficulty expressing anger or sadness in symbolic modes through language or pretend-play. A number of related deficits may impede their development, such as difficulty concentrating and attending to tasks, memory deficits that prevent them from integrating new material and relating it to old memories, and difficulty in abstracting and classifying.[29] Other children, in spite of adequate attachment relationships and capacity for symbolization, have difficulty controlling their impulses and complying with rules and have failed to internalize standards and rules of the environment. Many of these children have lacked structure and limits within their home environments. Measuring a number of relevant capacities within the child will help in identification of the principal areas of difficulty and planning of the most appropriate treatment strategies. Table 3 lists a

Table 3. Assessment of aggressive preschoolers

The child	Parent–child interaction	Parents and family	Social and environmental factors
Attachment disorders		Personality structure of parent(s)	
Capacity for relatedness	Reinforcement of positive behaviors	Psychiatric history and current	Socioeconomic level Housing
Caretaking history including separations	Response to negative behaviors	disorders Degree of depression	Social supports Family stressors Employment
Attachment measure of reunion with caregiver	Encouragement during teaching tasks Ways to deal with	Attachment to parents Alcoholism of	Educational level Isolation or degree of integration into
Level of self-esteem	anger Encouragement of play	parents Who the child represents for	extended family or community
	Encouragement of	the parents	
Neurologic and physiologic problems	verbal expression of feelings	Family Family dysfunction Marital relation-	
Developmental level		ship	
Neurologic assessment			
Difficulties with symbolization			
Language development			
Level of pretend play			
Cognitive controls			
Ability to commu-nicate about feelings and intent			

number of factors that should be determined by formal tests, observations, or interviews. (See Table 2 for a list of assessment instruments.)

Parent–child interactions and relationships

A growing number of studies of aggressive children have concluded that the quality of the caregiver–child relationship is critical in determining the child's continuing tendency to express anger through physical modes.[10,30–36] Observation of the parent–child interaction in the home and in the playroom is a critical component of any assessment. Observation should record the caregiver's responsiveness to positive behavior and his or her style of disciplining negative behavior. The contingency and consistency of these responses should also be noted, as aggressive children have frequently experienced indiscriminate caregiving and poor limit setting, with discipline swinging drastically from severe to lenient without reference to the behavior of the child.[37–40] Other components that should be observed are the caregiver's ability to teach the child task completion, to negotiate separations, and to encourage pretend-play and verbal expression of feelings. Perhaps most critical is an estimation of the quality of caregiver–child interaction and the degrees of acceptance or rejection, hostility or affection, positive or negative affect, and the sensitivity of the caregiver's reactions to the child's cues. Table 3 lists the critical components of this part of the assessment, and Table 2 lists some appropriate tests and observation schedules.

Personality structure and marital relationship of the parents

Hyperaggression in older children has been associated in research with a number of personality characteristics in their parent(s). For example, increased incidence of paternal criminality, antisocial personality development, violence, and substance abuse has frequently been found.[41–44] There is also evidence of linkage between disruptive behavior disorders in children and a range of related disorders in their mothers, who are more likely to exhibit criminal behavior, have depression,[45,46] and exhibit alcoholism or hysteria.[47] Recently, researchers have been assessing the internal attachment models or early memories of parents and have found that negative or insecure models are frequently associated with a high incidence of violent outbursts in their children.[27,28] A linkage with other, more subtle personality difficulties has not been as clearly identified, but they undoubtedly have a significant impact on the warmth and appropriateness of the interactions and care that parents provide for their children. Obtaining data on the parents is frequently difficult, especially in regard to such sensitive issues as the use of alcohol and the number of criminal convictions. Unstructured interviews with parents concerning their own experience of being parented will usually yield rich data with which to begin to understand their resistance to or difficulty in providing adequate nurturing.

Severe family dysfunction and conflictual marital relationships have been listed in a number of studies as factors contributing to antisocial behavior in children.[1,4,32,48] These influences are particularly strong if the child has witnessed violence between caregivers. Family dysfunction has its strongest influence in the early years through its impact on the primary caregivers, and it may affect the degree of energy and emotional availability that parents can provide in their relationships with their children. A listing of the areas that should be assessed under this category are listed in Table 3, and suggested assessment instruments are listed in Table 2.

Social and environmental factors

Studies have consistently found a strong correlation between lower socioeconomic class and aggression and conduct disorders.[49] Offord et al[1] found a similarly strong link between being on welfare and living in subsidized housing and aggression. However, it would seem that the link is not a direct one and is mediated by family discord and disturbed family function. A growing literature describes the impact of the lack of social support systems and family stressors, such as unemployment and poverty, on the development of children; these factors must be considered in any assessment of hyperaggressive preschoolers.

Case reports

Two clinical vignettes can illustrate how important assessment can be in determining the optimal manner of intervention.

J. Smith, aged 3 years, was referred for treatment by his mother because he had been expelled from the day-care center. Complaints included excessive tantrums and hurting of other children, inattention, and noncompliance. Teachers at the day-care center described Mr. and Mrs. Smith as angry and belligerent people who had failed to comply with requests made by day-care staff in regard to J.'s behavior. They felt that Mr. Smith was excessively punitive. Although assessment showed that the parents were at a loss to know how to manage J., it also showed that they cared for him deeply and struggled to provide adequate limit setting and positive interactions. J. was obviously unable to control his own impulses and to fantasize or play imaginatively. Testing showed that his verbal intelligence quotient (IQ) was 35 points lower than his performance IQ and that he was constantly distracted by external stimuli, showing little ability to concentrate on the task at hand. A narrow focus on the parents would almost certainly have ignored and missed the important characteristics of the child that contributed to the symptoms of aggression and that needed specialized treatment strategies.

A. Jones, aged 3 years, was referred by his mother, a single parent, who saw him as a "monster" who threw furniture around and who constantly terrorized his older sister and neighborhood children. Mrs. Jones's description of A. at referral suggested that he was a hyperactive child with significant delays in a number of developmental areas. In early observations, A. appeared to be a child with excessive anger and a sense of being rejected within his family. In addition, during early interviews and observations with A., Mrs. Jones revealed her own abuse by her father and exhusband and her fear that A. was the same as "the other males in her life." Her descriptions of A. at birth and how he looked at her—as if "he was out to get me"—suggested severe difficulties in her perception of her child and in her expectations of all males as aggressive and uncontrollable. In this case, a narrow focus on either the child or the mother's parenting techniques would have missed attitudes and fears within the mother that significantly affected her interaction with A. and, consequently, the development of the symptoms of aggression.

TREATMENT OF AGGRESSIVE PRESCHOOLERS

Assessment will frequently identify deficits and difficulties at several points within the transacting system: within the child, parents, interactions, and social milieu. The choice of points of entry at which to begin treatment may not necessarily influence the eventual therapeutic outcome[50]; however, it is critical that data from clinical assessment should determine which therapeutic modalities should be used. Unfortunately, in reality, the choice is often determined by the availability of resources and the theoretic orientation favored by the therapist assigned to the case. In the past, this tendency may have contributed to the lack of success reported in many studies of treatment efficacy with this population.

The child

By the time hyperaggressive preschoolers are identified for treatment, their symptoms are usually extreme. In many cases, therefore, it will be necessary to provide treatment for the child, individually or in a group setting such as a nursery school, in addition to treatment aimed at the parents or family.

When the child is evaluated individually, assessment will determine the most appropriate focus of the treatment and whether it should commence with nondirective play therapy or should incorporate sessions that carry out highly directive teaching of missing cognitive structures and interactional capacities. Children who lack the capacity for abstraction and symbolic play may need very structured activities that teach a number of cognitive capacities before they can benefit from more nondirective play therapy.[29,51] Alternatively, the two types of intervention may be used simultaneously by one or two therapists. J., the first child described above, was a clear example of the need for training of cognitive capacities before using play therapy. Observations in play sessions showed his inability to move beyond destructive play themes and his difficulty with integrating interpretations of his style of play. Testing revealed delays in body control, attention deficits, and difficulties in moving between fantasy or memories and reality. It was necessary to begin treatment with extensive teaching of these capacities before using more nondirective play techniques.

Children whose aggression is related to insecure attachment and who show developmentally appropriate cognitive capacities are likely to benefit from the therapeutic relationship, understanding, and acceptance that can be provided during play sessions. If traumatization, particularly through abuse, has contributed to the attachment disorder, the bringing to the surface of frightening unconscious material and reexperiencing it in a less threatening setting will free the child to begin to integrate painful memories with new positive experiences. For children who lack internalized controls, the limits that can be provided in play therapy sessions can help them understand and integrate the standards, rules, and expectations of the external world.

Aggressive children present a number of challenges in play therapy, as they frequently spend the majority of time in early sessions trying to run out of the room, hiding from the therapist, and engaging in games characteristic of children younger than themselves. It is as if they missed these games and the accompanying assurance of interaction during infancy.[52] Again, angry feelings and destructive themes typically dominate their play, even as they begin to settle down and begin to be able to use pretend-play and to integrate interpretations. It frequently takes months of sessions before the child can fully engage in more interactive and richer symbolic play. However, play therapy may provide children with a unique opportunity to deal with previously unconscious material, and at the same time may improve their capacity for imaginative play, sequential memory, and delay of impulsive behavior. A few studies[53-56] have shown these kind of improvements in aggressive preschoolers when play sessions have been used as part of the treatment strategy.

The child in group settings

In group settings, aggressive children present an enormous challenge; they may end up getting expelled or burning out day-care workers, thus setting themselves up for a response that is consistent with their history of perceived rejection by their parents. In some communities, therapeutic or specialized settings may be available that use a small group, structure, and skillful interventions by specially trained teachers. In an evaluative study of these settings, Anderson et al[57] reported that, although some aggressive, resistant children improve, they do not usually do as well as children whose symptoms are more internalized. More recently, integrative approaches have been used in preschool settings where the children who have been acting out are provided with one-to-one intervention but remain in normal day-care settings. If the child is not too disturbed or if a specialized setting or one-to-one intervener is not available and the child is placed in a normal day-care setting, it is important that someone be identified as the child's "special person," who can provide the one-to-one attention that the child needs when he or she loses control and acts out. In the case of J. presented earlier, support and training by the therapist of an identified day-care worker contributed significantly to the success of the outcome.

The day-care setting for aggressive toddlers should have a well-structured, organized, and predictable program. Because aggressive and impulsive children are frequently unable to anticipate or avoid situations that cause them excessive stress, planning for these events should be provided and coping strategies taught to the child by day-care workers. Observations of the child will provide information on those activities that seem to produce the most anxiety, stress, and potential for losing control. Similarly, the special worker will need to observe closely to catch the child being good and should show interest in and acknowledgement of positive behavior.

With many aggressive children, physical exercise and movement can be encouraged as legitimate ways to express frustration, and they are an important part of any treatment program. The teacher should also use a number of ritualized, stylized, simple social games and action songs that serve to improve language and provide positive, exciting, repetitive experiences of interaction for the young child. Helping the children to verbalize their feelings, label them, and communicate thoughts and anxieties through play and language are critical. Pretend-play and social interactions with peers should be encouraged and expanded. When the child does lose control, it will be essential for the identified special worker to help the child verbalize his or her feelings and to encourage him or her to experiment with other strategies to express anger. Demonstration of role playing and problem solving can be an excellent technique to facilitate an increased capacity to control impulses and to delay acting-out behaviors. Self-esteem can be improved by providing the child with experiences of success by breaking activities down into very small units and rewarding achievements in those units. Because many hyperaggressive preschoolers lack a sense of their own competence and of trust in others, it may take several months or even years before they can consistently control their acting-out behavior, particularly in a group setting.

The parent–child interaction

Traditionally, interventions with aggressive children have concentrated on teaching the parents new techniques to use in disciplining their children. This has included showing the parents how to provide rewards for positive behaviors and how to ignore acting-out behaviors. More recently, a number of parenting programs are also emphasizing the critical importance of encouraging parents to have positive experiences with their children and to set aside times for play and family meetings and outings. Others have encouraged the use of play by parents.[55–59] Parents are encouraged to act like "therapists" and to allow their children to initiate activities and to choose play themes. They learn how to follow the children's lead, to be sensitive to their cues, and to reflect verbally what the children are saying and doing. Beyond these positive interactions, parents must be helped to develop successful strategies to structure home life to discourage acting-out behavior and to bring their children's aggressive behavior under control. Frequently, parents will need concrete help in the home as well as modeling of techniques before they are able to reduce aggressive behavior. These techniques may include a time-out or the imposition of a particular consequence, but it is critical that the parents use the chosen techniques consistently and over a long period of time. In both cases presented in this article, extensive in-home parent training was necessary, in addition to other treatment strategies.

The teaching of these techniques and principles can vary from family to family. Some parents will prefer in-home assistance, others prefer to come to an office setting, and others find a group setting with other parents the most beneficial. Therapists may choose a structured parenting program, such as those developed by Barkley,[58] Eyberg and Matarazzo,[59] Forehand and McMahon,[60] and Webster-Stratton et al,[61] (and: Speltz ML, Beike B, Cantor J, Wittuner L. 1985. Unpublished manuscript) or a nonstructured program that allows the group leader more flexibility in addressing the specific concerns that parents may bring to the group sessions.

The parents

In some instances, parents appear unable to utilize and follow a parenting training course or other suggestions about parenting, and it becomes evident that unconscious metaphors and the parents' internal representation of their children are impeding the process of behavioral change. The case report of A. Jones and his mother illustrates this type of situation. These parents, who often are from extremely high-risk and multiproblem families of origin, may themselves have experienced severe traumatization and losses in childhood. Frequently, the child represents to the parent someone in his or her past, and the parent is unable to see and understand the individuality of the child and his behavior. Similarly, a marital problem may be acted out in interactions with the child. A number of approaches may be used in such cases, including attempts to change the interactive behaviors, individual therapy for the parents, or family therapy. In all efforts, the emphasis will be on increasing the parents' ability to see their children in new ways and to enable them to support one another in providing both positive interactions and limit setting for their children.[62] Painful past experiences must usually be resolved before new information and strategies can be integrated into parent–child interactions.

Social and environmental factors

If a number of social stressors are impinging on the family, concrete help in obtaining adequate housing, employment, and food can be necessary before treatment can begin. In the case of Mrs. Jones, an important part of the treatment program was helping her to find adequate employment and housing in addition to individual therapy. These supportive functions are used in many infant mental health programs and are designed to ease the stresses on the family system, rather than to remove or improve behavioral difficulties. They will therefore not be dealt with in this article.

•   •   •

There is little doubt that many hyperaggressive preschoolers become conduct-disordered children and adolescents. It seems critical to identify these children early and to provide specialized services to them before they enter school and begin to repeat the same cycle of rejection they experienced at home. As well, patterns of behavior and internalized representations become more difficult to change as the child passes beyond the preschool years. It is likely that, although treatment can in some instances be short-term, in many of the more serious cases, long-term and intensive services similar to those made available to autistic and developmentally delayed children are needed.[63,64] Because of the complexity of both the diagnosis and treatment of these children, input from a number of professionals with a wide range of expertise is necessary. In determining the choice of treatment, it is essential to consider the developmental capacities of the child, the internal representations of the parents, the family dynamics, and the wider social system. Research has not as yet confirmed the efficacy of this prescriptive approach in treating aggressive preschoolers. However, its success is well documented in a number of early intervention studies.[16,62] Further research is necessary to compare various treatment strategies and to facilitate clearer identification of the critical components of each. To date, research has not clearly delineated the developmental pathway to the control of aggression or elucidated the reasons for the development of hyperaggression in preschoolers. Only greater understanding of the pathways to the optimal development of self-regulatory systems will enable us to carry out more informed diagnostic decision making and to intervene in the most cost-effective way.

Certainly, identifying aggressive toddlers and providing mental health services to them and their parents present an enormous challenge. The families are often highly resistant to treatment unless they are in crisis, and many communities may lack programs and trained professionals to identify and treat these children. It is critical that a number of professional disciplines develop treatment strategies for helping aggressive preschoolers and integrate those strategies into their current clinical practice. For example, we need to train physical therapists to assess and teach children with delayed cognitive capacities, public health nurses to teach parenting techniques, and occupational therapists and day-care teachers to provide play experiences for these children. The screening of whole populations of preschoolers for these types of difficulties and the utilization of the current health care system to provide treatment for this population present a difficult challenge. It is one that must be faced, however, or we are likely to continue to see rising crime rates and an increasing incidence of abuse and family violence.[62]

REFERENCES

1. Offord D, Alder R, Boyle M. Prevalence and sociodemographic correlates of conduct disorder. *Am J Soc Psychiatry.* 1986;4(4):272–278.

2. Rutter M, Cox A, Tupling C, Berger M, Yule N. Attainment and adjustment in two geographic areas. I—The prevalence of psychiatric disorders. *Br J Psychiatry.* 1975;126:493–509.

3. Rutter M, Tizard J, Whitmore K. *Education, Health and Behavior.* London: Longman, 1970.

4. Rosen BM, Bahn AK, Kramer M. Demographic and diagnostic characteristics of psychiatric clinic patients in the U.S.A. *Am J Orthopsychiatry.* 1964;34:455–468.

5. Olweus D. Stability of aggressive reaction patterns in males: A review. *Psychol Bull.* 1979;86:852–875.

6. Kelso J, Stewart M. Factors which predict the persistence of aggressive conduct disorder. *J Child Psychol Psychiatry.* 1986;27(1):77–86.

7. Offord DR, Reitsma-Street M. Problems of studying antisocial behaviour. *Psychiatr Dev.* 1983;2:207–224.

8. Robins LN. *Deviant Children Grown Up.* Baltimore, Md: Williams & Wilkins, 1966.

9. Robins LN. Epidemiological approaches to natural history research: Anti-social disorders in children. *J Am Acad Child Psychiatry.* 1981;20:566–580.

10. Campbell S. *Family characteristics and child behavior as precursors of externalizing symptomatology at school entry.* Presented at Biennial Meeting of the Society for Research in Child Development; April 25–28, 1985; Toronto, Ontario, Canada. ERIC document ED 262871.

11. Campbell S, Ewing L, Breaux A, Szumowski E. Parent-referred problem three-year-olds: Follow-up at school entry. *J Child Psychol Psychiatry.* 1986;27:473–488.

12. Morris H, Escoll P, Wexler R. Aggressive behavior disorders of childhood: A follow-up study. *Am J Psychiatry.* 1956;112:991–997.

13. Rose S, Rose S, Feldman J. Stability of behavior problems in very young children. *Dev Psychopathol.* 1989;1:5–19.

14. Kazdin AE. *Treatment of Antisocial Behavior in Children and Adolescents.* Homewood, Ill: Darsey Press, 1985.

15. Gould R. *Child Studies Through Fantasy.* New York: Quadrangle/The New York Times Book Co., 1972.

16. Greenspan SI. *Psychopathology and Adaptation in Infancy and Early Childhood.* New York: International Universities Press, 1981.

17. Gould R. Studies of aggression in early childhood: Patterns of attachment and efficacy. *Psychoanal Inquiry.* 1982;2(1):21–52.

18. Parens H. *The Development of Aggression in Early Childhood.* New York: Jason Aronson, 1979.

19. Sroufe LA. Infant-caregiver attachment and patterns of adaptation in preschool: The roots of maladaptation and competence. *Minn Symp Child Psychol.* 1983;16:41–81.

20. Provence S, Lipton R. *Infants in Institutions.* New York: International Universities Press, 1962.

21. Brinich PM. Aggression in early childhood: Joint treatment of children and parents. *Psychoanal Study Child.* 1984;39:493–508.

22. Downey TW. Within the pleasure principle: Child analytic perspectives on aggression. *Psychoanal Study Child.* 1984;39:101–136.

23. Redl F. *Children Who Hate.* New York: Free Press of Glencoe, 1951.

24. Harris R. Relationship between EEG abnormality and aggressive and anti-social behavior—a critical appraisal. In: Hersov LA, Berger M, eds. *Aggression and Anti-Social Behaviour in Childhood and Adolescence.* Oxford: Pergamon Press, 1978.

25. Hill D. Notes and criticisms. Weekend conference on psychopathic personality. *Br J Delinquency.* 1951;2:154.

26. Lewis D, Pincus J, Lovely R, Spitzor E, Moy E. Biopsychosocial characteristics of matched samples of delinquents and non-delinquents. *J Am Acad Child Adolesc Psychiatry.* 1987;26(5):744–752.

27. Main M, Kaplan N. Security in infancy, childhood and adulthood: A move to the level of representation. *Monogr Soc Res Child Dev.* 1985;50(1–2):66–102.

28. Main M, Solomon J. Discovery of an insecure-disorganized/disoriented attachment pattern. In: Braselton TB, Yogman MW, eds. *Affective Development in Infancy.* Norwood, NJ: Ablex, 1986.

29. Santostefano S. *Cognitive Control Therapy with Children and Adolescents.* New York: Pergamon Press, 1985.

30. Bates J, Bayles K. Attachment and the development of behavior problems. In: Belsky J, Nezworske T, eds. *Clinical Implications of Attachment.* Hillsdale, NJ: Erlbaum, 1988.

31. George C, Main M. Social interactions of young abused children: Approach, avoidance, and aggression. *Child Dev.* 1979;50:306–318.

32. Lefkowitz M, Eron L, Walder L, Huesmann LR. *Growing Up To Be Violent. A Longitudinal Study of the Development of Aggression.* New York: Pergamon Press, 1977.

33. Lowrey LG. Personality distortion and early institutional care. *Am J Orthopsychiatry.* 1940;10:576–586.

34. Olweus D. Familial and temperamental determinants of aggressive behaviour in adolescent boys: A causal analysis. *Dev Psychol.* 1980;16:644–660.

35. Walsh A, Beyer J. Violent crime, sociopathy and love deprivation among adolescent delinquents. *Adolescence.* 1987;22(87):705–717.

36. Dumas JE, Wahler RG. Indiscriminate mothering as a contextual factor in aggressive-oppositional child behavior: "Damned if you do and damned if you don't." *J Abnorm Psychol.* 1985;13(1): 1–17.

37. Eron LD, Walder L, Lefkowitz M. *Learning of Aggression in Children.* Boston: Little, Brown, 1971.

38. Patterson GR. The aggressive child: Victim and architect of a coercive system. In: Mash E, Hamerlynck A, Handy L, eds. *Behavior Modification and Families. Theory and Research.* New York: Bruner/Mazel, 1976.

39. Parke RDS, Dewar JL. Schedule of punishment and reinforcement of punishment in children. *Dev Psychol.* 1972;7:266–269.

40. Sawin D, Parke R. Empathy and fear as mediators of resistance-to-deviation in children. *Merrill Palmer Q.* 1980;26(2):123–133.

41. Behar D, Steart M. Aggressive conduct disorder: The influence of social class, sex and age on the clinical picture. *J Child Psychol Psychiatry.* 1984;25(1):119–124.

42. Stewart MA, DeBlois CS, Cummings C. Psychiatric disorders in the parents of hyperactive boys and those with conduct disorder. *J Child Psychol Psychiatry.* 1979;21:283–292.

43. Stewart M, DeBlois CS. Wife abuse among families attending a child psychiatry clinic. *J Am Acad Child Psychiatry.* 1981;20:845–862.

44. Stewart M, DeBlois C. Father-son resemblances in aggressive and anti-social behaviour. *Br J Psychiatry.* 1983;142:78–84.

45. Cicchetti D, Abei JL. Early precursors of later depression: An organizational perspective. In: Lipsitt L, Rovee-Collier C, eds. *Advances in Infancy Research,* vol 4. NJ: Ablex, 1986.

46. Zahn-Waxler C, Cummings E, McKnew D, Radke-Yarrow M. Altruism, aggression and social interactions in young children with manic depressive parents. *Child Dev.* 1984;55:112–122.

47. Cantwell DP. Psychiatric illness in the families of hyperactive children. *Arch Gen Psychiatry.* 1972;27:414–417.

48. Bettleheim B. *Love is Not Enough.* New York: Free Press of Glencoe, 1952.

49. Maccoby EE, Gibbs PK. Methods of childrearing in two social classes. In: Martin WE, Stendler CB, eds. *Readings in Child Development.* New York: Harcourt, Brace, 1954.

50. Stern-Bruschweiler N, Stern D. A model for conceptualizing the role of the mother's representational world in various mother-infant therapies. *Inf Ment Health J.* 1989;10(3):142–156.

51. Santostefano S. *A Biodevelopmental Approach to Clinical Child Psychology: Cognitive Controls and Cognitive Control Therapy.* New York: Wiley, 1978.

52. Willock B. *The Hyperaggressive Child: A Biopsychological Model.* Ann Arbor, Mich., University of Michigan: 1980. Dissertation.

53. Udwin O. Imaginative play training as an intervention method with institutionalized preschool children. *Br J Educ Psychol.* 1983,53:32–39.

54. Vaughn S, Ridley CA, Bullock DC. Interpersonal problem-solving skills, training with aggressive young children. *J Appl Dev Psychol.* 1984;5:213–223.

55. Eyberg SM, Robinson EA. Parent-child interaction training: Effects on family functioning. *J Clin Child Psychol.* 1982;11:130–137.

56. Denny B, Hillard D. Documentation of change in problem behaviors among anxious and hostile-aggressive children enrolled in a therapeutic preschool program. *Child Psychiatry Hum Dev.* 1981;11(4): 232–240.

57. Anderson DR, Long A, Leathrs E, DeDenny B, Allard D. Documentation of change in problem behaviors among anxious and hostile-aggressive children enrolled in a therapeutic preschool program. *Child Psychiatry Hum Dev.* 1981:11(4):232–240.

58. Barkley RA. *Defiant Children: A Clinician's Manual.* New York: Guilford, 1987.

59. Eyberg SM, Matarazzo RG. Training parents as therapists: A comparison between individual parent-child interaction training and parent group didactic training. *J Clin Psychol.* 1980;36:492–499.

60. Forehand R, McMahon R. *Helping the Noncompliant Child: A Clinician's Guide to Parent Training.* New York: Guilford, 1981.

61. Webster-Stratton C, Kolpacoff M, Hollinsworth M. Self-administered video-tape therapy for families with problem children: Comparison of two cost-effective treatments and a control group. *J Consult Clin Psychol.* 1988;56(4):558–566.

62. Fraiberg S. *Clinical Issues in Infant Mental Health.* New York: Basic Books, 1980.

63. Schorr L. *Within Our Reach: Breaking the Cycle of Disadvantage.* New York: Anchor Press, 1988.

64. Kazdin A. Treatment of antisocial behavior in children: Current status and future directions. *Psycholog Bull.* 1987;102:187–203.

Treatment of sensory, emotional, and attentional problems in regulatory disordered infants

Georgia A. DeGangi, PhD
Director of Cecil and Ida Green
  Research and Training Institute
Reginald S. Lourie Center for Infants
  and Young Children
Rockville, Maryland
Clinical Instructor
Department of Pediatrics
Georgetown University
Washington, DC

Polly Craft, MD
Medical Director
Reginald S. Lourie Center for Infants
  and Young Children

Joan Castellan, MS
Pediatric Nurse and Child
  Development Specialist
Reginald S. Lourie Center for Infants
  and Young Children

INFANTS WITH constitutional difficulties present parents and professionals with a unique and complex challenge. Fussy or difficult infants have been described as experiencing disorders of regulation that involve persistent difficulties including emotional regulation, arousal and state control, and sensory modulation.[1] (See "Assessment of sensory, emotional, and attentional problems in regulatory disordered infants: Part 1."[2]) The symptoms commonly exhibited by the regulatory disordered infant include fussiness, irritability, poor self-calming, intolerance for change, and a hyperalert state of arousal. Frequently these infants are hypersensitive to sensory stimuli, including auditory, tactile, visual, and vestibular stimulation.[1] Attentional problems including distractibility, poor impulse control, and an inability to sustain attention are often present. These constitutional difficulties affect not only the way in which the child interacts with the world and processes information, but also the way in which others, particularly parents, interact with the child.

A comprehensive and integrated model of assessment and treatment is needed to address the constitutional problems of the regulatory disordered child and the impact of these problems on the family and the parent–child dyad. An expanded model of treatment is proposed that includes the following components:

- parent guidance that focuses on management of sleep, feeding, and behaviors in the home environment;
- child-centered activity that fosters healthy parent–child interactions within the context of play; and
- sensory integrative therapy techniques that promote organized attention, adaptive behaviors, and normalized responses to sensory experiences.

The various components of the family-centered treatment approach are provided by a multidisciplinary team consisting of a child psychiatrist, pediatric

Inf Young Children 1991; 3(3): 9–19

nurse, early childhood specialist, speech and language pathologist, occupational therapist, and developmental psychologist. Two members of the team meet directly with the family during the therapeutic process, while the other team members serve as consultants to the primary clinicians. The parent guidance, child-centered activity, and sensory integrative therapy techniques are blended together in treatment, with primary emphasis on meeting the immediate needs of both the parent and child.

In this article, the family-centered approach is described as it is applied to regulatory disordered infants. The elements of parent guidance are presented with examples of typical problems. Child-centered activity and sensory integrative therapy techniques are discussed in their application to infants with sensory, emotional, and attentional deficits. Lastly, a case example is presented that incorporates the various elements of the treatment approach.

THE FAMILY-CENTERED APPROACH

Recent legislation and current research on family involvement in a child's therapy program point to the value of a family-centered approach to intervention. In this approach, play is increasingly recognized by professionals as an important medium through which parents can address the special needs of their child. Play is viewed as the arena in which children learn and practice new skills with the people most important to them.[3] Recent research suggests that when parents realize a sense of empowerment in making decisions, stress and depression may be reduced and their sense of competence may be increased.[4] Clinicians become consultants to the parents in this collaborative model of helping, and the parents' abilities are acknowledged with respect and confidence.[5]

Children who are fussy, irritable, and demanding are extremely challenging for parents. Often parents cope by developing interaction patterns of understimulation or overstimulation. For example, parents who must often soothe and regulate their distressed child may find that they tend to retreat or shrink from interaction when their child is happy and to be content to "not rock the boat." In the case of the highly distractible child who appears to seek constant novelty, the parents may exacerbate the problem by presenting many activities or toys to their child to try to keep him or her happy.

In the family-centered approach, it is important to recognize the stress that coping with a difficult child places on the family. Parents often experience sleep deprivation and, as a result, have little reserve for coping with an irritable child. Many parents report that babysitters cannot cope with the child's difficult behaviors, which compounds feelings of entrapment. Marital tension may be heightened as the parents feel overwhelmed by the problems of the fussy and difficult child or make accommodations that interfere with their own lives (eg, infant sleeping in parents' bed). In some cases, the father distances himself from the family, working long hours to avoid a hectic home life and a constantly screaming infant. The danger of child abuse is very real.

An adequate support system is necessary to help a family cope with a difficult situation. More and more parents find that they have no extended family in their geographic area and, as a result, have no one to help them or to provide respite. Play groups have become an alternative support system for many families; however, many fussy infants cannot tolerate being in a play group situation, thus removing this option for the parent. Additionally, many parents take their children to baby gym or swim classes, but these activities often are too stimulating for the regulatory disordered child. As a result, many parents feel even more isolated and removed from the typical activities in which parents engage with their children. Sometimes parents who try such options feel stigmatized by other parents because their child appears to be out of control.

Parents often experience depression secondary to coping with the demands of parenting a fussy infant. Many mothers report feelings of inadequacy when normal parenting skills do not seem to work with their child. First-time parents often confuse their child's constitutional difficulties with parental inexperience, which exacerbates depression or feelings of helplessness. These feelings are compounded when the infant rejects being held and cuddled because of hypersensitivities to touch. Sometimes the parents learn to avoid sensorimotor activities that provoke their child's hypersensitive responses. For example, if the child dislikes swings and playground equipment because of extreme fearfulness of movement in space, a protective mother may guide her child away from movement activities. In some cases, the parents may experience similar hypersensitivities, compounding their responses to an infant who shares constitutional difficulties.

In summary, a family-centered approach focuses on parental concerns, family stresses in coping with the difficult child, adaptive and maladaptive parent–child interaction patterns, and parental depression or marital conflicts secondary to the child's constitutional difficulties. These issues may be addressed directly through parent guidance and the child-centered activity.

PARENT GUIDANCE

Parental guidance is an important component of the family-centered approach. It provides parents with emotional support in coping with their difficult child and aids them in developing effective strategies to set limits and manage their child's sleep, self-calming, and feeding problems. Although parent guidance is individualized, a variety of self-help books often is used to help parents manage specific problems such as sleep or dietary problems.[6-8] Although the relationship between food allergies and behaviors is controversial, the possibility of food allergies should be explored for those children who do not respond to behavioral management techniques. For example, it was recently reported that a significant number of infants who did not respond to behavioral techniques for sleeplessness did respond to a hypoallergenic diet that eliminated all milk products.[9]

When therapy is initiated, the clinician seeks to help the parents understand their child's behaviors and how they as parents do and should respond when the behaviors occur. The clinician and parents discuss what techniques have already been tried to determine which ones have worked. The clinician should ascertain whether parental inexperience or mismanagement of behaviors exacerbates the child's regulatory difficulties or whether the father and mother manage their child's difficult behaviors differently.

Parent guidance takes the form of a working dialogue with each parent to develop the best match between the parent's concerns, the family life style, and management techniques. Major emphasis is placed on developing problem-solving strategies that enable parents to gain insight into their child and themselves. For example, some parents may realize that they are overcontrolling and cannot tolerate their child's overly active and loud behaviors, such parents can be assisted in developing strategies to help their child organize behaviors before they become uncontrollable while providing opportunities for normal active exploration. Parent guidance blends the principles of behavioral management, supportive therapy, practical management techniques, and sensory integrative treatment.

The most common areas that are addressed in parent guidance include sleep management, consoling the crying infant, managing feeding difficulties, and focusing the distractible child's attention in play. Some of the techniques employed in each of these areas are discussed.

Sleep management

Sleep disorders in children are very complex. For this reason, clinicians must obtain a detailed history to ascertain the type of sleep disorder. Some infants trained to awaken for a middle-of-the-night feeding or trained to awaken by parents who remove their baby from the crib when he or she cries in the night develop sleep disorders. Some infants develop fearfulness when waking in the night that may be related to separation anxiety; in most infants, this problem resolves after 1 month. Other sleep problems are physiologically based. The child may have difficulty inhibiting a high state of arousal to fall asleep and stay asleep for any length of time. Such children often are very active during their sleep. A review of the common types of sleep problems in infants is presented by Schmitt.[10]

Before developing a sleep management program, a 3-day record should be obtained detailing the child's normal routines, feeding schedule, and sleep activity. In addition to the sleep record, it is important to determine what techniques may or may not have been effective in getting the infant to fall asleep and stay asleep. Parents who experience anxiety, problems with separation, a low threshold for tolerating distress in their infant will consequently pick up the infant every time he or she wakes and cries. Another problem evolves when parents who are desperate for sleep invite their wakeful infant into their own bed and then find it difficult to reestablish the infant's crib as a place to fall asleep and stay asleep.

Most infants beyond 6 months of age who experience sleep disturbances respond to behavioral management and the introduction of appropriate sleep routines.[11] Before change is introduced, the sleep activity record should be examined for a hint of a biological pattern, which will provide the basis for improved timing of sleep–wake activities over 24 hours. Parents should establish nighttime routines that prepare the infant for sleep through soothing and calming activities such as massage, lullabies, books, and prayers. Infants should be put to bed in an awake state so that they learn how to put themselves to sleep. Periods of crying are permitted for 5, 10, and 15 minutes the first night, gradually increasing to 20, 25, and 30 minutes on the fourth night. Most children acclimate to this program within the first week. Some parents require enormous support in this effort, while others are eager to solve the problem once they have a plan of action. Parents should be reassured that their infant may need to cry for 5 to 15 minutes before falling asleep and that this is not atypical.

One strategy for helping parents manage their infant's sleep problems is to use sensory inhibition to diminish arousal prior to bedtime. Linear movement activities (eg, forward-back and head-to-toe rocking, swinging) are calming and serve to inhibit the reticular activating system via the vestibular system. Firm deep pressure is a technique that helps to inhibit a hypersensitive tactile system. Swaddling, baby massage, or activities that provide firm touch help to dampen a highly aroused tactile system. Dimming of the lights, soft rhythmic music, white noise (eg, recording of ocean waves), and focused visual activities (eg, simple pictures) are also suggested.

Some infants need additional help to fall or stay asleep once placed in bed. A crib cradle (ie, a hammock swing designed for the crib), a vibrating mattress, a warm blanket from the dryer, or a water bed mattress help to further soothe the overaroused infant. A nest of pillows piled around the infant provides neutral warmth and a sense of tactile security. (Care should be taken to avoid suffocation in small infants.) Infants who startle themselves awake sometimes are helped by tightening a sheet over their body to prevent the extraneous arm and leg movements that wake them in the night. White noise audiotapes can help decrease arousal through habituation to a constant auditory stimulus. Whenever sensory inhibitory techniques are used, parents need to learn to observe carefully to determine what helps their infant to modulate the level of arousal and to fall asleep.

Consoling the crying infant

When an infant is inconsolable, it is important to determine if medical problems are the primary reason for the crying (eg, colic, chronic ear infections, reflux, severe allergies). When medical problems have been ruled out, inconsolability may be related to hypersensitivity to environmental stimulation and incapacity to self-calm. In some cases, a crying infant may be responding to tensions in the parent, who may handle the infant briskly or in ways that are not conducive to calming. Excessive crying may be related to separation issues, and for some infants it may occur whenever changes are introduced in the everyday routine or activity. A complete history of when and where crying occurs and how long it lasts is useful in determining the causes of the behavior.

A common problem confronting the parent who is trying to console a crying infant is a tendency to become frantic when consistent efforts do not seem to work. The mother may rock vigorously forward and back for a short period of time, then shift to swinging the infant in the air when crying resumes. Parents often fear that other caregivers may abuse their overly distressed baby and therefore never leave their child with other caregivers, even when respite is sorely needed. When parents must cope with an infant who cries more than 2 hours per day, respite is necessary to help parents restore their capacity to deal with their overly fussy infant.

It is important to help the parents remain calm while trying to console their crying infant and to use a technique long enough to evaluate its effectiveness. Sometimes the parent's tolerance of the infant's fussiness is very low. Parents of very young infants should be encouraged to calm their crying infant, but once the infant reaches 5 or 6 months, he or she should be given the opportunity to self-calm and to learn to resolve frustration with support and encouragement from the parents. When crying persists beyond 5 or 10 minutes even after the parents have encouraged the infant to self-calm (eg, presenting the infant's pacifier or a favorite toy), the parents should seek to calm their infant by holding and rocking or other effective means.

An important goal of parent guidance is to help the infant to develop self-calming. Some infants quiet when looking at or listening to something novel. Others respond better when helped to organize their own movements. Often parents need to begin by providing sensory inhibition through firm, deep pressure and linear movement. Bringing the hands to midline, touching the palms to body parts, or helping the child suck on his or her own fingers are simple ways that this may be accomplished. After developing self-calming behaviors, the infant should be helped to use these or his or her own rather than continuing to be organized and calmed by others.

Managing feeding difficulties

Feeding difficulties may be related to constitutional factors, such as sensory hypersensitivities, oral-motor problems, and food allergies, or to preexisting or resultant problems in the parent–child relationship. The most common behavioral feeding problems reported by parents include refusal to eat, difficulty remaining seated in the high chair, extreme food preference, and food throwing. Many parents become concerned about their child's nutritional intake when these behaviors occur and find themselves feeding the child out of the high chair while he or she plays or takes a bath to ensure that the child is eating enough.

Strong food preferences are not uncommon, and often parents report that the child spits out foods with unfamiliar textures. Hypersensitivity to touch in the mouth may be the problem. Often, parents can desensitize these hypersensitivities by allowing the child to move firm, plastic-bristled toothbrushes or electric toothbrushes around in the mouth. Firm, brisk scrubbing around the lips and on the gums sometimes helps to desensitize the mouth.

An extensive food history and examination of behaviors is important to determine if food intolerances or food allergies may be causing the child's irritability and sleep problem. A strong preference for one food may indicate a food allergy. Pediatricians are becoming increasingly aware that the antigen-antibody explanation of food allergies does not always explain allergic reactions in children. The foods, chemicals, or drugs that cause allergic-like reactions work directly on the basophil and/or mast cells of the immune system with no antibody intervention whatsoever. Everything in the environment—food, air, water, places of play—triggers unpleasant reactions in some children.

Focusing the distractible child's attention in play

A common problem associated with hyperarousal is an intense need for novelty and new stimulation, with an accompanying short attention span. A hyperaroused child goes from one toy to another and does not play with any toy long enough to develop a toy preference. Parents find themselves planning many activities in a given day to keep their child occupied or providing many toys to the child. An interactional style of overstimulation often develops. If a mother observes her child's short attention span and need for novelty and responds by offering another toy to keep her child content, the child never goes back to the same toy to learn the many different ways to play with the same toy.

In parent guidance, the home environment can be restructured so that only a few toys are available to the child at a given time. A child with a short attention span often responds well to having a small enclosed space that becomes his or her special play area. A small pup tent, for example, filled with a nest of soft pillows or a small play house may help the child to contain his or her activity level within a confined area.

CHILD-CENTERED ACTIVITY

Addressing the emotional aspects of the interactive difficulties that exist between the regulatory disordered infant and the parents is central for treatment. The authors' approach focuses on using the inner resources of both child and parent. Using an experiential model, child-centered activity is a form of infant psychotherapy that is adapted to the sensorimotor phase of development.[12,13] Greenspan and Greenspan[14] called the elements and mechanics of child-centered activity for parents "floor time." The parent is taught to provide regular daily 15- to 30-minute sessions of focused, nonjudgmental attention. During this time, the child is the initiator of all the play, and the parent is the interested observer and facilitator. The child is encouraged to engage in activities that he or she enjoys. The child's attention span and activity level dictate the direction that the play takes, rather than an imposed structure or specific task demand presented by an adult. The environment is organized to make toys and materials available that will promote sensorimotor development in a safe area where no "nos" or prohibitions apply. Because the child sets the agenda for the play, activities tend to be at or slightly above the child's capabilities (eg, a young toddler learning to walk may enjoy testing his or her balance by walking up and down a ramp). In addition, extrinsic reinforcement, such as praise, is deemphasized. Instead, the parent reflects on the child's expressivity through expanding on facial gestures, affect, or language cues.

The underpinnings of this approach lie in the view that play is the medium by which a child learns, rather than direct instruction and skills training, and that children learn best when actively engaged in the presence of a loving parent. As the child becomes the initiator of an interaction, intrinsic motivation and active participation in interactions and explorations are enhanced. The child experiences the parents' encouragement to act on his or her interests, which enhances the child's feelings of success, competence, and control. As a result, the child learns to develop internal control and to plan or map how to engage in explorations with the environment and interactions with others. Since the parent reflects on what the child is doing in this approach by following the child's lead, the child gains a sense of becoming effective in interacting with the parent, an important skill that empowers the child's ego development.

Through the medium of child-centered activity, parents become more sensitized to their child's behavioral style, developmental needs, and interests. For a child with significant sensory disturbances, this learning has far-reaching implications. For example, the infant with tactile hypersensitivities may avoid handling textured objects, reject new food textures, and experience physical discomfort when touched by others. Because of the underlying tactile hypersensitivities, the infant may exhibit difficulty in manipulating small objects, feeding, and playing with peers. In treatment, the mother may set out several types of tactile exploration toys (eg, a large bin of styrofoam chips with many interesting toy figures buried inside the bin) during the time designated for child-centered activity. She will wait and watch the child as he or she approaches the materials, facilitating exploration by taking turns. In this way, the child learns to explore the materials on his or her own terms, taking in only as much tactile information as his or her nervous system can handle. Aggressive behaviors may be channeled appropriately by providing the child with toys such as heavy push carts that he or she can lift and move or large spongy balls and bats that can be thrown and hit with. These types of activities also serve to desensitize the child's overly sensitive tactile system.

The child-centered activity approach has been applied by individuals in several disciplines to accomplish different goals. Speech and language therapists have used this approach to achieve balanced interactions between an adult and child through turn-taking. The child initiates an action, and the adult imitates the action or vocalization or responds by continuing the child's topic. This turn-taking exchange may continue for a number of turns with variations in responses occurring with each turn. Turn-taking not only serves to facilitate communication, but also assists in increasing attention to tasks. This approach has been used successfully with mentally retarded and developmentally delayed children.[15,16]

The ultimate goals of the child-centered activity for an infant are to
- provide the child with focused, nonjudgmental attention from the parent;
- facilitate self-initiation and problem-solving by the child;
- develop intentionality, motivation, curiosity, and exploration;
- promote sustained and focused attention;
- refine the child's signal giving;
- enhance mastery of sensorimotor developmental challenges through the context of play; and
- broaden the repertoire of parent–infant interactions.

The goals for a parent are to
- develop better signal reading of their child's cues and needs,
- become more responsive to their child, allowing him or her to take the lead in the interaction,
- develop a sense of parental competence as a facilitator rather than a director of their child's activity,
- take pleasure in their child in a totally nonprohibitive setting,
- appreciate their child's intrinsic drive for mastery and the various ways in which it is manifested, and
- change the parent's internal representation of himself or herself and the child to that of a competent parent and a competent child.

Because the focus of the approach is on mastery for both parent and child, it is a highly positive and reinforcing experience for both parent and child. Preconceived notions that a child must be taught in order to learn are challenged, particularly for the parent who perceives the child as less competent than his or her peers. The parent's weaknesses and limitations are not considered detrimental to the treatment process; however, these difficulties and problems must be addressed. Some parents may not be able to embrace this approach. Child centered activity expects parents to take a role that may be anxiety provoking; parents with obsessive or rigid parenting styles may find the more reflective and responsive style of interaction difficult. If it can be mastered, child-centered activity may help parents develop less rigid patterns of interaction and allow for an expanded repertoire of parent behaviors that later enhance mental health. Child-centered activity is a natural foundation for listening skills.

Mothers with mild to moderate depression often find that child-centered activity provides them with something to work on with their child. Once a depressed mother begins to see progress in her child's behaviors, she often feels improved self-esteem and effectiveness as a parent. In addition, different parental styles (eg, protective, prohibitive, competitive, facilitatory) are recognized and are useful to clinicians as they try to sensitize parents in how they relate to and manage their infant.

SENSORY INTEGRATIVE THERAPY APPROACH

Sensory integrative therapy, developed by Ayres,[17,18] provides a foundation for children experiencing sensory processing and attentional deficits. This therapy is provided within the context of child-centered activity and parent guidance. Treatment techniques already described for desensitizing the hyperreactive child, organizing sustained attention and purposeful activity, and promoting self-calming and modulation of arousal states are derived from the sensory integrative treatment approach.

The underlying premise of sensory integrative theory is that the ability of the central nervous system to take in, sort out, and interrelate information received from the environment is necessary to allow for purposeful, goal-directed responses. The major principle underlying sensory integrative treatment is the improvement of an individual's ability to organize and process sensory input provided during meaningful events, thus allowing for an adaptive response to the environment. A child's ability to actively experience sensations while simultaneously engaging in self-directed, purposeful motor activity is essential to intervention. Sensory integrative therapy facilitates an individual's ability to make adaptive responses to environmental stimuli, and these responses facilitate organization in the central nervous system by providing sensory feedback about a goal-directed event.

Self-directed and self-initiated actions differentially enhance central nervous system function and maturation.[19] In essence, such approaches as child-centered activity allow a child to develop automatic functions of better self-organization and control. The theoretical mechanism is the somatomotor adaptive response which, by definition, is an appropriate motor response to a sensory event, the internal feedback of which enhances central nervous system organization and maturation and the process of organizing a response to a sensory environmental demand.[20]

CASE EXAMPLE

T was referred to the Reginald S. Lourie Center for Infants and Young Children by his parents at 17 months of age because of extreme irritability. He was a white male living at home with his mother (30 years old) and father (34 years old). T's father was an attorney, and his mother was a homemaker and the primary caretaker. When T was seen for the initial interview session, he was crying uncontrollably in his mother's arms in the waiting room. He cried throughout most of the session, only occasionally quieting down and wandering about to explore the toys in the office. Even when spoken to softly, he began to cry again inconsolably.

His mother's chief concerns were that T was different from other infants and that he was very hard to handle. T was recognized as different soon after birth. On his second day of life, a nurse from the newborn nursery approached his mother and said, "You are going to have to do something about T. He's keeping all the other babies awake." When he came home from the hospital, he slept approximately 12 out of 24 hours and screamed most of the time he was awake.

A pediatrician diagnosed T as having "colic" and prescribed Donnatal when he was 4 weeks old. Neither parent wanted their infant to be medicated, so the mother instead got a referral to a nurse practitioner. She explained that T was very easily overstimulated, even by such things as faces, lights, and noises. The nurse recommended decreasing stimulation by such measures as holding him facing away from herself when feeding and soundproofing his sleep environment.

T's mother reported that during his first year, he had otitis about five times, which was then used as the explanation for his persistent crankiness. There was no evidence of chronic ear pathology, and the remainder of his medical history was negative. He had good weight gain on breastfeeding, but was weaned at 3 1/2 months of age because he kicked and punched, which the mother interpreted as his way of fighting being held. Once on bottle feedings, he slept through the night. He now goes to bed, gets to sleep, sleeps through the night, and awakens in the morning on his own.

The mother tried to return to working part-time when he was 3 1/2 months old. He was placed in a family daycare, where he was the only child. The caretaker described T as "sensitive" and often reported to his mother that he was "cranky all day." T's mother gave up going to work when the babysitter decided to take in other children. Although the mother wanted to return to work, she felt that T's fussiness could cause a caretaker who did not love him to abuse him. The parents had a limited support system to provide respite. The father's sister and brother-in-law watched T briefly on a few occasions, and a teenage babysitter was employed for a few hours in the daytime.

T's mother reported that she felt that his father had always been able to soothe him a little better than she could and that he was T's preferred person. Whenever she felt frustrated with T, she gave him to her husband. Her husband pointed out to her several times that she was acting irritable and tense with the child. The mother admitted having a great personal struggle with her current feelings about T, which she described as being doubtful of her capacity to be a mother. She reported having felt this way even before T was born, mainly because she felt she lacked the experience to be a good mother. She felt publicly embarrassed by his unsoothable crying and had experienced an exacerbation of psychophysiological problems since his birth (the recurrence of a spastic colon).

Diagnostic workup

Developmental testing using the *Bayley Scales of Infant Development,*[21] mental scale, was conducted, and T was found to be functioning at age level. Despite his age-appropriate cognitive level of functioning, he exhibited evidence of an expressive language delay but appeared to have no receptive language difficulties. In addition, he was unable to sit and play with toys, had difficulty initiating planned and purposeful actions, and demonstrated slow processing time during attentional tasks. On the *Test of Sensory Functions in Infants,*[22] T demonstrated severe hypersensitivities to touch and movement and an inability to plan simple motor actions in response to a sensory stimulus (ie, textured mitt placed on his foot). His primary interests were in gross motor tasks, but he had recently begun to like to look at pictures and magazines. His balance was poor, with falling, instability, and low muscle tone in his movement quality. Overall, T exhibited delays in expressive language and in balance and muscle tone; was hypersensitive to touch, sound, and movement; and had attentional difficulties. In spite of his mother's feelings of inadequacy, at every meeting she was gentle and supportive of him. On parent–child interaction measures, the mother was observed to be understimulating and at times nonparticipating and withdrawn when T played quietly. Mother's interactions centered around helping T to obtain a toy out of reach or to introduce a new toy when he became fussy or distracted. No symbolic play or reciprocal interactions were observed. T's manipulation of toys was highly stereotypic and imma-ture for his age (eg, taking toys in and out of box, shaking and banging).

Treatment process

The treatment sessions focused on decreasing the tension between T and his mother and, in the context of unpressured play with her, on developing initiative, reciprocal interactions, purposeful manipulation of toys, regulation of mood state, and desensitized responses to touch and movement. During the child-centered ac-tivity, T spent a considerable amount of time lifting heavy push carts and pound-ing and pushing them on the floor, thus providing himself with heavy propriocep-tive input and desensitizing his responses to loud noises. His mother discovered that when she gently imitated him, his pleasure and length of playing time in-creased. In the first week of treatment, T's mother was encouraged to allow him to play in a large bin of styrofoam chips and to explore textured objects (eg, slinky and rough hairbrushes), tactile activities that T soon began to crave.

Within a short period of time, T developed a strong interest in interacting with both his parents. He appeared to derive enormous pleasure out of reciprocal inter-actions with them. His father began to attend the sessions and shared more excite-ment and involvement with his son. By the third week of treatment, T's crying behavior was greatly diminished. The critical break appeared to occur once T was able to express himself through gestures and could tolerate touch, sounds, and movement. T became much less reliant on his close-to-the-ground positions, in-cluding the W-sitting posture, using trunk rotation in transitional movements, and he fell much less often when walking. Moreover, he became very interested in looking at pictures and wanted to know the names of everything.

After a short-term intervention, T was referred to the local public school's es-tablished early identification program for enrollment. Furthermore, individualized speech and language therapy and occupational therapy were indicated. As T im-proved, his mother began to talk about the contribution her self-doubts and depres-sion had made to their difficulties. The exacerbation of her irritable bowel symp-toms led her to begin individual psychotherapy.

•   •   •

Within the family-centered intervention approach, a combination of parent guidance, child-centered activity, and sensory integrative therapy techniques are needed to address the complex needs of the difficult child. Parent guidance tech-niques provide parents with specific management techniques to handle their child's sleep and feeding problems and irritability. Child-centered activity, a form of infant psychotherapy, enhances parent–child interactions and facilitates self-initiation, sustain attention, purposeful behavior, and communication in the child.

Sensory integrative therapy techniques are integrated within the context of parent guidance and child-centered activity to normalize the child's responses to sensory stimulation, modulate arousal and state control, and promote organized, adaptive responses during play and everyday activities. Systematic research is needed to examine the effectiveness of the specific treatment approaches and its value as an integrated model for children with regulatory disorders.

REFERENCES

1. DeGangi GA, Greenspan SI. The development of sensory functioning in infants. *Phys Occup Ther Pediatr.* 1988;8(3):21–33.

2. DeGangi GA. Assessment of sensory, emotional, and attentional problems in regulatory disordered infants: Part I. *Inf Young Children.* 1991;3(3):1–8.

3. Schaaf RC, Mulrooney LL. Occupational therapy in early intervention: A family-centered approach. *Am J Occup Ther.* 1989;43:745–754.

4. Friedrich WN, Cohen DS, Wilturner LT. Specific beliefs as moderator variables in maternal coping with mental retardation. *Children's Health Care: J Assoc Care Children's Health.* 1988;17:40–44.

5. Dunst CJ, Trivette CM, Davis M, Cornwell J. Enabling and empowering families of children with health impairments. *Children's Health Care: J Assoc Care Children's Health.* 1988;17:71–81.

6. Daws D. *Through the Night: Helping Parents and Sleepless Infants.* London, England: Free Association Books; 1989.

7. Rapp D. *The Impossible Child.* Tacoma, Wash: Sciences Press; 1986.

8. Sears W. *The Fussy Baby.* Franklin Park, Ill: Le Leche League International; 1985.

9. Kahn A, Mozin MJ, Rebuffat E, Sottiaux M, Muller MF. Milk intolerance in children with persistent sleeplessness. *Pediatrics.* 1989;84: 595–603.

10. Schmitt BD. The prevention of sleep problems and colic. *Prev Primary Care.* 1986;33:763–774.

11. Ferber R. Diagnosis and treatment of sleep disorders in children. *Pediatr Basics.* 1984;39:7–14.

12. Ostrov K, Dowling J, Wesner DO, Johnson FK. Maternal styles in infant psychotherapy: Treatment and research implications. *Inf Ment Health J.* 1982;3:162–173.

13. Mahrer AR, Levinson JR, Fine S. Infant psychotherapy: Theory, research, and practice. *Psychother Theory, Res Pract.* 1976;13:131–140.

14. Greenspan SI, Greenspan NT. *The Essential Partnership.* New York, NY: Viking; 1989.

15. Mahooney G. Enhancing the developmental competence of handicapped infants. In: Marfo K, ed. *Parent-Child Interaction and Developmental Disabilities: Theory, Research, and Intervention.* Westport, Conn: Praeger; 1988.

16. Mahooney G, Powell A. Modifying parent–child interaction: Enhancing the development of handicapped children. *J Spec Educ.* 1988 ;22:82–96.

17. Ayres AJ. *Sensory Integration and the Child.* Los Angeles, Calif: Western Psychological Services; 1979.

18. Ayres AJ. *Sensory Integration and Learning Disorders.* Los Angeles, Calif. Western Psychological Services; 1972.

19. Kandel ER, Schwart JH. *Principles of Neural Science.* 2nd ed. New York, NY: Elsevier; 1985.

20. Clark FA, Mailloux S, Parham D. Sensory integration and learning disabilities. In: Pratt PN, Allen AS, eds. *Occupational Therapy for Children.* New York, Mosby; 1985.

21. Bayley N. *Bayley Scales of Infant Development.* New York, NY: Psychological Corporation; 1969.

22. DeGangi GA, Greenspan SI. *Test of Sensory Functions in Infants.* Los Angeles, Calif: Western Psychological Services; 1989.

Early intervention and stimulation of the hospitalized preterm infant

Yvette Blanchard, MS, PT
Candidate for Doctorate in
    Therapeutic Studies
Sargent College of Allied Health
    Professions
Boston University
Boston, Massachusetts

THE EFFECTS OF an impoverished versus an enriched environment on the brain have been relatively well studied and documented in the animal.[1] Manipulation of the environment has been shown to lead to changes in the gross weight of the brain, changes in the weight and thickness of the cerebral cortex, and microscopic changes in cell density and relative proportions of different neurons.[1] Neurochemical and physiologic changes have also been demonstrated. Unfortunately, relatively little is known about the possible influence of the environment on the human brain, as manipulation of the environment is under strict ethical ruling, and direct methods of quantifying changes in the brain are very limited.

This avenue of research is of particular interest to those involved in the care of the hospitalized preterm infant. There is some debate over the type of intervention and stimulation these infants should be provided with, but it is believed by most that stimulation and intervention in some form are beneficial.[2] Controversies exist over what is appropriate stimulation and how it should be offered to these infants. There are two general approaches to the administration of stimulation. In one of them, different modalities of sensory stimulations are provided separately, with little attention paid to the overall environment and actual overall sensory experience of the hospitalized preterm infant.[3-18] In the other one, primary attention is directed at structuring the environment and caregiving procedures based on the detailed evaluation of the infant's level of functioning in the extrauterine environment.[19-22] In the latter approach, appropriate sensory stimulations are provided. They are, however, offered through the whole approach of care instead of being administered in an isolated fashion. The purposes of this article are to review the literature and discuss the research conducted in support of both approaches and to highlight the contribution that each body of research has made to the field of early intervention and stimulation of the hospitalized preterm infant.

SENSORY STIMULATION OF THE PRETERM INFANT

Since the 1960s, numerous studies have been conducted to examine the effects of sensory stimulation on the hospitalized preterm infant. The majority of the stimulation programs offered tactile stimulations alone or sometimes accompanied with other forms of sensory stimulations, such as auditory, visual, olfactory, vestibular, and proprioceptive.[3-18] In most of these studies, the need for interven-

Inf Young Children 1991; 4(2): 76–84
© 1991 Aspen Publishers, Inc.

tion was based on the belief that the preterm infant was in a state of sensory deprivation within the extrauterine environment. Stimulations that were either absent or diminished had to be supplemented.[8,9,13,15-18] This assumed state of deprivation could be related to isolation in the incubator,[15,16,23] to the lack of stimulations that would normally be present in utero,[5,9,13,24,25] or to the comparison of the stimulation received by a fullterm newborn infant.[25] The goal of these stimulation programs was to compensate for the lack of stimulation or to provide an enriched environment to promote development. In either case, additional stimulation was believed to be beneficial.

Following this first upsurge in stimulation programs for the preterm infant, some researchers[23,26] started questioning the validity of the assumption on sensory deprivation. Cornell and Gottfried[23] argued that systematic observation of the actual level of stimulation was needed before any generalization could be made on the degree of stimulation offered to the preterm infant. Subsequent observations of the neonatal care unit showed that levels of noise and light far exceeding established norms were present constantly with no diurnal cycles.[26] Lawson and colleagues[26] concluded that the preterm infant's environment provided sensory overstimulation rather than sensory deprivation.

Gottfried[27] generally agreed with this perspective. His findings, however, showed that not only is the quantity of stimulation an area of concern but so is the quality of sensory experience. For example, tactile stimulation was observed to be most often associated with therapeutic intervention, with or without pain, and very infrequently to offer comfort.[27-29] Sensory stimulations were shown to be most often experienced in an isolated fashion. For example, the infant would be touched but would not see the person touching him or her.[26] As well, very little contingency was noted between the expression of a need and its satisfaction. Stimulations were not contingent on behaviors displayed by the infants. New types of sensory stimulation programs, temporally patterned or contingent to behaviors of the infant, then made their appearance.[3,11] But until now, it seems that very little research on sensory stimulation has been conducted from the perspective of overstimulation rather than deprivation.

Most studies on sensory stimulation do not provide a theoretical model for the effects sought. Only the most recent studies reporting the effects of tactile stimulation on weight gain do so.[4,6,12] Their models are based on animal research conducted with rats,[30] in which separation of the rat pup from its mother was shown to cause a decline in brain and heart ornithine decarboxylase activity and a decrease in the secretion of serum growth hormone. These detrimental effects were subsequently shown to be specifically associated with the absence of tactile stimulation as provided by the mother during licking[31] (also: Pauk J, Kuhn CM, Field TM, Schanberg SM. Written communication. April 1987). Further studies showed that these ill effects can be prevented by providing the deprived rat pups with heavy stroking, while light stroking showed no effects.[31]

On the same continuum, most of the studies on sensory stimulation do not report compelling theoretical rationales for selecting any specific type, quantity, or patterning of stimulation. Blanchard and colleagues[4] have attempted to do so in their study examining the effects of tactile stimulation on physical growth and the risk of hypoxemia in preterm infants. Based on information gathered from many sources—namely, animal studies[31] (also: Pauk J, Kuhn CM, Field TM, Schanberg SM.) observations by Umphred and McCormack,[32] preliminary trials with three preterm infants, and consultation with experienced therapists in neonatology[4,33]—a pressure of 10 in of water was selected as the amount of tactile pressure administered to the stimulated infants. The tactile stimulations were applied via an air-filled cushion connected to a sphygmomanometer that enabled quantification and control of and visual feedback on the amount of pressure applied. Their results, however, showed no effects of tactile stimulation on physical growth. Further research is still needed to determine the specific patterning of administration and the optimal amount of tactile pressure to apply for beneficial effects on physical growth.

In the last decade, there has been some concern over the effects of handling and of different therapeutic interventions on the preterm infant's blood oxygen saturation levels. Chest physical therapy, social interaction, and other common interventions including suctioning, diaper and position change, physical examination, venous and arterial puncture, injection, feeding, and recording of vital signs were identified as possible causes of hypoxemia.[34,35] If common therapeutic interventions can affect the level of blood oxygenation, so could sensory stimulation programs. Only one study[4] reported the use of an oximeter to control for possible hypoxemic episodes during tactile stimulation. The results showed no risk of hypoxemia but showed that oxygenation during stimulation was better with the infants in the prone position compared to those in the supine position. These authors recommend caution in generalizing these findings to all preterm infants, as their sample included healthy and relatively robust preterm infants. More research of this type is needed to ascertain that there are no risks involved for the stimulated infants.

The studies conducted on the effects of sensory stimulation differ on the type, quantity, and total duration of sensory stimulation administered, on the samples of preterm infants studied, and on the variables chosen to measure their effects. Given their diversity, it is very difficult to come to any general conclusion regarding their effects on the development of preterm infants, but general tendencies can be reported.

Weight gain has been the most common dependent variable. Results, however, are varied and sometimes even contradictory. Some studies report higher weight gain for the infants stimulated with tactile and kinesthetic stimulation[6,12,13,15,17,18] or with vestibular and auditory stimulation,[9] while other studies report no weight gain following tactile stimulation[4,8,16] or multisensory stimulation, including visual, tactile, kinesthetic, and auditory stimulation.[10] Unlike other studies, the study on tactile stimulations conducted by Solkoff and colleagues[17] included follow-up testing. Their findings showed that the weight-gain advantage previously observed for stimulated infants was lost after 6 weeks of life. When evaluating weight gain, caloric intake should also be considered. Even if results were not positive following multisensory stimulation (visual, tactile, kinesthetic, auditory), Leib and colleagues[10] noted that their stimulated infants had a lower caloric intake for a weight gain equal to that of the control group. White and Labarba[18] noted that the infants provided with tactile or kinesthetic stimulations ingested more calories per meal but had fewer meals per day than the control group. However, Field and colleagues[6] reported a higher weight gain for infants stimulated with tactile or kinesthetic stimulations, in spite of an equal daily caloric intake with the control group. It would be worthwhile to elucidate the mechanisms underlying these findings. These mechanisms could, for example, explain if weight gain is related to an increased caloric intake, a calmer state, or a slower metabolism that favors a decreased need for calories.

Effects of sensory stimulation on psychomotor development have also been measured by testing with the following instruments: the Bayley Scales of Mental Development,[36] the Brazelton Neonatal Assessment Scale,[37] Cattell,[38] Denver,[39] and Gesell.[40] In the majority of these studies, positive results on psychomotor development were reported.[3,10,13,17] Only one study[8] reported no difference between groups. Since consistently positive results have been observed on psychomotor development, it is suggested that this measure be considered in future studies. As the psychomotor acquisitions in the first months of life of preterm infants are limited, it is also suggested that a follow-up observation be performed.

In summary, the effects of sensory stimulation on the development of preterm infants are varied: sometimes even contradictory, but very often positive. From this review of literature, it is possible to put forth a few recommendations. The selection of an outcome measure should be made according to the type of effect sought, either specific (weight gain) or general (psychomotor development),[24] and should be supported by a theoretical framework. Cornell and Gottfried[23] recommend the use of multiple outcome measures, as this would increase the possibility of finding an area of development in which beneficial effects would be observed. The long-term benefits of this approach to stimulation also need to be determined. Even though it could be agreed that stimulation is beneficial to preterm infants, many questions remain to be answered: For whom and at what conceptional age should these be applied? How and at what intervals should they be administered? And for what purpose?[41]

INDIVIDUALIZED BEHAVIORAL AND ENVIRONMENTAL CARE

The approach presented in this section is based on the work of Als and colleagues.[19,42] Before a description of how this model is clinically applied, its theoretical background and rationale for intervention will be presented.

A high proportion of prematurely born children show some degree of learning disabilities that cannot be clearly related to the presence of known cerebral insult.[43] As an explanation, it has been suggested that the premature birth itself might have important consequences for the subsequent neural development,[44] suggesting that some of the medical and developmental problems resulting from premature birth arise from the immature organism's difficulty in adapting to the caregiving environment outside the womb.[45,46] It has thus been proposed that the management of the preterm infant's sensory environment, including physical and social aspects, be given as much importance as the management of his or her medical care.

The developmental changes occurring in the brain between 26 and 40 weeks of gestation are considerable and correspond to the beginning of the most active period of organizational events.[47] During this period, progressive enrichment of dendritic and axonal plexus accompanied by the appearance of synaptic connections, development of neurofibrils, and increase in the size of the Nissl substance of cells is believed to occur. The brain as designed and constructed by the genome is not fully developed at birth.[48] According to Spinelli,[48] full configuration of the brain takes place after birth and is guided by stimuli, information, and challenges that originate in and are specific to a particular environment. The preterm infant is faced very early on with the task of achieving homeostasis in the presence of a large variety of stimuli-taxing systems that may not be ready for stimulation. Yet, stimuli have to be given to help the infant achieve or maintain homeostasis, interact with the environment, and configure his or her neural and mental potential. These stimuli should be controlled and matched as closely as possible to the needs and actual level of sensory integration capacities of the preterm infant.[48] At an early stage of development, Parmelee[49] proposed that it is more important to protect the preterm infant from as many stimuli as possible in order to stabilize biologic homeostasis, than it is to provide additional stimulation.

As all areas of the brain are intimately interrelated, damage in one area may have an impact on other areas,[45] resulting in subtle neuromotor abnormalities,[50] learning disabilities, and behavior problems.[51-53] Direct or indirect brain insults are seen as the consequence of a mismatch between the extrauterine environment and the capacity of the central nervous system of the preterm infant, adapted for an intrauterine existence, to adapt to the extrauterine environment.[45] To adequately support and protect the preterm infant from such insults, detailed evaluations of the extrauterine environment and of the capacity of the central nervous system to deal with such an environment need to be documented. It is believed that the environment of the preterm infant should be monitored and controlled as a whole and that sensory modalities need not be separated.[44,46,54,55]

Als's hypothetical synactive theory of the development of the preterm infant describes the gradual unfolding of the infant's intraorganism subsystems: the autonomic system that assures the organism's baseline functioning; the motor system with its recognizable flexor posture and limb and trunk movements; the state organizational system with its distinct states of consciousness; and the attentional/interactive system with its differentiated awake state that is capable of elaborated affective and cognitive receptivity and activity.[19] A fifth subsystem, the self-regulatory subsystem, is found within each of the other four subsystems. These subsystems support and influence each other (thus the term synactive) in an environment appropriate for their development.[19] The underlying theoretical formulation of the synactive theory is based on the biphasic balancing between the approach to appropriate stimulation and the defense against or avoidance of inappropriate stimulation.[56] Infants will display stress or defense behaviors and self-regulatory or approach behaviors in each of the subsystems.

These behaviors provide the avenue by which the brain and its functioning in the extrauterine environment will be assessed.[40] Using the Neonatal Individualized Developmental Care and Assessment Program (NIDCAP) (Als H. 1984. Unpublished data), the detailed observation of these behaviors will be made when the infant is quiet and undisturbed and during any type of therapeutic manipulation. The thresholds from balanced modulated functioning to stressed and disorganized functioning will be documented for each of the subsystems. From these observations, a profile of the current behavioral and developmental instability and fragility and the current regulatory strengths can be established[45] (also: Als H. 1984. Unpublished data).

From the synactive theoretical model and systematic NIDCAP observation of the infant's behaviors, an individualized care plan can be implemented. Based on the behaviors displayed by each infant, the immediate environment and the caregiving therapeutic approach will be adapted to the infant's specific needs.[19,42] The goals of these adaptations will be to facilitate the reduction of stress behaviors and the increase of self-regulatory behaviors. The approach is highly individualized and adapted to each infant's specific level of maturation. When appropriate, additional sensory stimulations are provided, but the administration, in terms of choice of modality or quantity, is not necessarily comparable between infants. As well, these sensory stimulations are provided through the whole structure of the environment and caregiving procedure (eg, tactile stimulation via swaddling), rather than through isolated administration by a clinician.

Other very important aspects of the approach of Als and colleagues are the role and direct involvement of the parents in the care of their premature infant. As the infant is seen as part of a family unit parents are involved from day 1 in the planning of the services and needs of their infant. The meanings of stress and self-regulatory signals are readily explained to each parent thereby facilitating their understanding of the infant's behaviors and their level of comfort when providing care for their infant. It has recently been documented that parents given the opportunity to observe their infant's behavioral capabilities during the Assessment of Preterm Infant Behavior (APIB) had more realistic perceptions of their infant, that fathers had less anxiety, and that mothers seemed more aware of their premature infant's attempt to shut out disturbing stimulation.[57]

The hypothesis that attention to the individual infant's behavioral cues leading to appropriate changes in their environment and care would result in the reduction of stress behaviors, the increase of specific self-regulatory behaviors, and improved medical developmental outcome, has been tested.[42] Significant differences between experimental and control groups have been shown. In terms of medical outcome, the experimental infants experienced significantly briefer stays on the respirator and in increased FiO_2 and showed significantly earlier breast or bottle feeding. Developmental outcome showed significantly better behavioral regulation scores on the APIB at 1 month after the estimated date of confinement (EDC),[58,59] significantly better mental and psychomotor developmental scores on the Bayley Scales at 3, 6, and 9 months post EDC, and significantly better behavioral regulation scores on the Kangaroo-Box Paradigm[42] at 9 months post-EDC.

A replication study has been conducted with a larger sample.[45] Significant differences between experimental and control infants were also shown. Experimental infants showed significantly shorter stays on the respirator, fewer days on supplemental oxygen, earlier breast or bottle feeding, improved average daily weight gain from birth to 42 weeks postconception age, a younger postconception age at discharge, a shorter hospital stay, and a lower incidence of intraventricular hemorrhage. The incidence of bronchopulmonary dysplasia was not different between these groups; however, the severity score (grades 0–3) was significantly lower in the experimental group. APIB scores at 2 weeks after due date and brain electrophysiologic functioning at the same date have also shown significant differences between groups, favoring the experimental infants.[60] These infants are currently being followed for long-term outcome.[45]

This developmental and highly individualized approach to the care of hospitalized preterm infants has been incorporated at Brigham and Women's Hospital (BWH) in Boston, Massachusetts, for over 10 years. Over time, observations of these infants have suggested that certain motor behaviors, specifically those involving extension, were noted less frequently. As well, if the goals of this care plan are met, it would be expected that preterm infants treated at BWH a few years after the approach was implemented would show increased approach behaviors and decreased avoidance behaviors when compared to an earlier, treated group of preterm infants. To test this hypothesis, Mouradian[61] compared the APIB scores of two groups of 20 preterm infants: a cohort of infants treated at BWH between 1978 and 1979 and a cohort of infants treated between 1982 and 1986. Of the 17 motor variables scored by the APIB, 7 showed significant differences between the two groups in which the 1982 to 1986 group showed decreased extensor motor patterns and increased flexor patterns. Of the 29 summary variables measured by the APIB, 8 showed significantly better scores for the 1982 to 1986 group. Six of these 8 summary variables indicated improved motor functioning, while the other 2 indicated improved state organization and increased behavioral organization.[61]

These results are very promising. Longitudinal follow-up will further determine the impact of this approach on later cognitive and psychomotor functioning. The intervention approach suggested by this model implies a complete change in the way care has traditionally been provided in the neonatal intensive and intermediate care units. Once established, this approach remains part of the routine of care. However, this endeavor is a tremendous challenge to the proponents of this approach and the primary caregivers.

•   •   •

This review shows that extensive work has been conducted by both groups advocating stimulation of and intervention for the preterm infant in the intensive or intermediate care unit. In the first approach presented, in which supplemental stimulation is prescribed, research has predominantly examined the effects of stimulation on the physical and psychomotor development of the infants. With some exceptions,[4,6,12] there is almost no theoretical background underlying these studies, and very little is known, even hypothetically, of the mechanisms triggered by such stimulation. The preterm infant is not perceived as an organism functioning in a context, but rather as an infant deprived of stimulation. Many questions and issues remain to be addressed in this area of research. However, it does provide very useful information on the sensitivity of the preterm infant to sensory and environmental stimuli. Even if research remains to be done on the specific protocol of administration of these stimulations, we do know that they somehow make a difference in the patterns of growth and development of preterm infants.

The approach to intervention of Als and colleagues is based on a detailed evaluation of each infant's level of functioning in the extrauterine environment through his or her behavioral responses to the environment and caregiving procedures.[42] It is based on a neurologic and developmental theoretical background that provides a rationale for intervention and a model for the effects sought. These researchers are also interested in examining the long-term effects of their approach, as they are currently still following these infants.[45] There is continuity to this research, a theory and paradigm provide a research context, and the results shown at this point have supported some aspects of their hypotheses. This approach is gaining increasing national recognition. Under the direction of Als, the National Collaborative Research Institute for Early Childhood Intervention is conducting nationwide research to further validate the approach and its effectiveness.

Research conducted in both groups has to be considered by those providing care for the preterm infant. It is important to know about the impact of sensory stimulation on development. It is also important to know about the infant's level of functioning in the extrauterine environment and to better understand the context within which stimulations can be applied. Fragile and medically compromised preterm infants need to be treated with such an outlook on their needs.

REFERENCES

1. Renner MJ, Rosenzweig MR. *Enriched and Impoverished Environments.* New York: Springer-Verlag, 1987.

2. Guzenhauser N. *Infant Stimulation: For Whom, What Kind, When, and How Much?.* Skillman, NJ: Johnson & Johnson Baby Products, 1987.

3. Barnard KE, Bee HL. The impact of temporally patterned stimulation on the development of preterm infants. *Child Dev.* 1983;54:1156–1167.

4. Blanchard Y, Pedneault M, Doray B. Effects of tactile stimulation on physical growth and hypoxemia in preterm infants. *Phys Occup Ther Pediatr.* 1991;11:37–52.

5. Edelman AH, Kraemer HC, Korner AF. Effects of compensatory movement stimulation on the sleepwake behavior of preterm infants. *J Am Acad Child Psychiatr.* 1982;21:555–559.

6. Field TM, Schanberg SM, Scafidi F, Bauer CR, Vega-Lahr N, Garcia R, et al. Tactile/kinesthetic stimulation effects on preterm neonates. *Pediatrics.* 1986;77:654–658.

7. Korner AF, Ruppel EM, Rho JM. Effects of waterbeds on the sleep and motility of theophylline treated preterm infants. *Pediatrics.* 1982;70:864–869.

8. Kramer M, Chamorro I, Green D, Knudtson F. Extra tactile stimulation on the premature infant. *Nurs Res.* 1975;24:324–333.

9. Kramer LI, Pierpont ME. Rocking waterbed and auditory stimuli to enhance growth of preterm infants. *J Pediatr.* 1976;88:297–299.

10. Leib SA, Benfield G, Guidubaldi J. Effects of early intervention and stimulation on the preterm infant. *Pediatrics.* 1980;66(1):83–90.

11. Pelletier JM, Short MA, Nelson NL. Immediate effects of waterbed flotation on approach and avoidance behaviors of premature infants. *Phys Occup Ther Pediatr.* 1985;5(2/3):81–92.

12. Scafidi F, Field T, Schanberg S, Bauer C, Vega-Lahr N, Garcia R, et al. Effects of tactile/kinesthetic stimulation on the clinical course and sleep/wake behavior of preterm infants. *Infant Behav Dev.* 1986;9:91–105.

13. Rice RD. Neurophysiological development in premature infants following stimulation. *Dev Psychol.* 1977;13:69–76.

14. Rose SA, Schmidt K, Riese ML, Bridger WH. Effects of prematurity and early intervention on responsivity to tactual stimuli: A comparison of preterm and full-term infants. *Child Dev.* 1980;51: 416–425.

15. Scarr-Salapatek S, Williams ML. The effects of early stimulation on low birthweight infants.

Child Dev. 1973;44:94–101.

16. Solkoff N, Matuszak D. Tactile stimulation and behavioral development among low birthweight infants. *Child Psychiatry Hum Dev.* 1975;6:33–37.

17. Solkoff N, Yaffe S, Weintraub D, Blase B. Effects of handling on the subsequent development of premature infants. *Dev Psychol.* 1969;1:765–768.

18. White JL, Labarba RC. The effects of tactile and kinesthetic stimulation on neonatal development in the premature infant. *Dev Psychol.* 1976;9:569–577.

19. Als H. A synactive model of neonatal behavioral organization: Framework for the assessment of neurobehavioral development in the premature infant and for support of infants and parents in the neonatal intensive care environment. *Phys Occup Ther Pediatr.* 1986;6(3/4):3–53.

20. Cole JG. Infant stimulation reexamined: An environmental and behavioral based approach. *Neonatal Network.* 1985;3:24–31.

21. Lawhon G. Management of stress in premature infants. In: Angelini JD, Whelan Knapp CM, Gibbs RM, eds. *Perinatal/Neonatal Nursing: A Clinical Handbook.* Boston: Blackwell, 1986.

22. VandenBerg KA. Behaviorally supportive care for the extremely premature infant. In: Gunderson LP, Kenner C, eds. *Care of the 24–25 Week Gestational Age Infant (Small Baby Protocol).* Petaluma, California: Neonatal Network, 1990.

23. Cornell EH, Gottfried AW. Intervention with premature human infants. *Child Dev.* 1976;47: 32–39.

24. Masi W. Supplemental stimulation of the premature infant. In: Field TM, ed. *Infants Born at Risk.* New York: SP Medical and Scientific Books, 1979.

25. Schaefer M, Hatcher RP, Barglow PD. Prematurity and infant stimulation: A review of research. *Child Psychiatry Hum Dev.* 1980;10:199–212.

26. Lawson K, Daum C, Turkewitz G. Environmental characteristics of a newborn intensive care unit. *Child Dev.* 1977;48:1633–1639.

27. Gottfried AW. Environment of newborn infant in special care units. In: Gottfried AW, Gaiter JL, eds. *Infant Stress Under Intensive Care.* Baltimore: University Park Press, 1985.

28. Blackbrun ST, Barnard KE. Analysis of caregiving events relating to preterm infants in the special care unit. In: Gottfried AW, Gaiter JL, eds. *Infant Stress Under Intensive Care.* Baltimore: University Park Press, 1985.

29. Newman LF. Social and sensory environment of low birthweight infants in a special care nursery. *J Nerv Ment Dis.* 1981;169:448–455.

30. Butler SR, Suskind MR, Schanberg SM. Maternal behavior as a regulator of polyamine biosynthesis in brain and heart of the developing rat pup. *Science.* 1978;199:445–446.

31. Evoniuk GE, Kuhn CM, Schanberg SM. The effect of tactile stimulation on serum growth hormone and tissue ornithine decarboxylase activity during maternal deprivation in rat pups. *Psychopharmacol.* 1979;3:363–370.

32. Umphred DA, McCormack GL. Classification of common facilitatory and inhibitory treatment techniques. In: Umphred DA, ed. *Neurological Rehabilitation.* St. Louis: Mosby, 1985.

33. Pedneault M, Blanchard Y, Lapalme S. Pression manuelle cutanee: Etude de fidelite inter et intratherapeutes. *Physio Canada.* 1990;42(3):130–135 .

34. Gorski PA, Hole WT, Leonard CH, Martin JA. Direct computer recording of premature infants and nursery care: Distress following two interventions. *Pediatrics.* 1983;72:198–202.

35. Long JG, Phillip AGS, Lucey JF. Excessive handling as a cause of hypoxemia. *Pediatrics.* 1980;65: 203–207.

36. Bayley N. *Manual for the Bayley Scales of Infant Development.* New York: Psychological Corp, 1969.

37. Brazelton TB. *Neonatal Behavioral Assessment Scale.* In: Clinics in Developmental Medicine, No. 50. Philadelphia: J.B. Lippincott, 1984.

38. Cattell P. *Infant Intelligence Scale.* New York: Psychological Corp, 1940.

39. Frankenburg WK, Dodds JB, Fandal AW, Kazuk E. *Denver Developmental Screening Test: Reference Manual.* Denver: Univ. Colorado Medical Center, 1975.

40. Ames LB, Gillepsie C, Haines J, Ilg FL. *The Gesell Institute's Child From One to Six: Evaluating the Behavior of the Preschool Child.* New York: Harper & Row; 1979.

41. Korner AF. Infant stimulation: Issues of theory and research. In: Gunzenhauser N, ed. *Infant Stimulation: For Whom, What Kind, When, and How Much?.* Skillman, NJ: Johnson & Johnson Baby Products, 1987 .

42. Als H, Lawhon G, Brown E, Gibes R, Duffy FH, McAnulty G, et al. Individualized, behavioral and environmental care for the very low birth weight preterm infant at high risk for bronchopulmonary dysplasia: Neonatal intensive care unit and developmental outcome. *Pediatrics.* 1986;78:1123–1132.

43. Cohen SE, Parmelee AH. Antecedents of school problems in children born preterm. *J Pediatr Psychol.* 1988;13(4):493–508.

44. Duffy FH, Mower G, Jensen F, Als H. Neural plasticity. A new frontier for infant development. In: Fitzgerald HE, Lester BM, Yogman MW, eds. *Theory and Research in Behavioral Pediatrics.* New York: Plenum Press, 1984.

45. Als H. Caring for the preterm infant. In: Bottos M, Brazelton TM, Ferrari A, Dalla Barba B, Zachello F, eds. *Neurological Lesions in Infancy: Early Diagnosis and Intervention.* Padoca, Italy: Liviana Editrice, 1989.

46. Gorski PA, Huntington L, Lewkowicz DJ. Handling preterm infants in hospital: Stimulating controversy about timing stimulation. In: Gunzenhauser N, ed. *Infant Stimulation. For Whom, What Kind, When, and How Much?.* Skillman, NJ: Johnson & Johnson Baby Products, 1987.

47. Volpe JJ. *Neurology of the Newborn.* Philadelphia: W.B. Saunders, 1987.

48. Spinelli DN. Plasticity triggering experiences, nature, and the dual genesis of brain structure and function. In: Gunzenhauser N, ed. *Infant Stimulation: For Whom, What Kind, When and How Much?.* Skillman, NJ: Johnson & Johnson Baby Products, 1987.

49. Parmelee AH. Sensory stimulation in the nursery: How much and when? *Dev Behav Pediatr.* 1985;6(5):242–243.

50. Goldson E. Bronchopulmonary dysplasia: Its relation to two-year developmental functioning in the very low birthweight infant. In: Field TM, ed. *Infants Born at Risk.* New York: Grune & Stratton, 1983.

51. Hertzig ME. Neurological "soft" signs in low birthweight children. *Dev Med Child Neurol.* 1981; 23:778–791.

52. Kitchen WH, Ryan MM, Rickards A, McDougall AB, Billson FA, Keir EH, et al. A longitudinal study of very low-birthweight infants. IV. An overview of performance at eight years of age. *Dev Med Child Neurol.* 1980;22:172–188.

53. Koops BL, Harmon RJ. Studies on longterm outcome in newborns with birthweight under 1500 grams. *Adv Behav Pediatr.* 1980;1:1–28.

54. Turkewitz G, Kenny PA. The role of developmental limitations of sensory input on sensory/perceptual organization. *Dev Behav Pediatr.* 198S;6(5):242–243.

55. Gottfried AW. Environmental manipulations in the neonatal period and assessment of their effects. In: Smeriglio VL, ed. *Newborn and Parents: Infant Care and Newborn Sensory Stimulation.* Hillsdale: Erlbaum, 1981.

56. Denny-Brown D. *The Cerebral Control of Movement.* Springfield, Ill.: Charles C Thomas, 1966.

57. Culp RE, Culp AM, Harmon RJ. A tool for educating parents about their premature infants. *Birth.* 1989;16(1):23–26.

58. Als H, Lester BM, Tronick E, Brazelton TB. Towards a research instrument for the assessment of preterm infants' behavior. In: Fitzgerald HE, Lester BM, Yogman MW, eds. *Theory and Research in Behavioral Pediatrics.* vol 1. New York: Plenum Press, 1982.

59. Als H, Lester BM, Tronick E, Brazelton TB. Manual for the assessment of preterm infants' behavior (APIB). In: Fitzgerald HE, Lester BM, Yogman MW, eds. *Theory and Research in Behavioral Pediatrics.* vol 1. New York: Plenum Press, 1982.

60. Als H. Continuity and consequences of behavior in preterm infants. In: von Euler C, Forssberg H, Lagercrantz H, eds. *Neurobiology of Early Infant Behavior.* Hampshire, England: Macmillan Press, 1989.

61. Mouradian L. N.I.C.U. care and motor functioning of preterm infants. *Newsl Boston Inst Dev Infants Parents.* 1989;8(1):5.

A partnership model for communicating with infants at risk

James D. MacDonald, PhD
Chief of Language
Associate Professor

Jennifer Y. Carroll, MA
Speech/Language Pathologist
The Nisonger Center
The Ohio State University
Columbus, Ohio

THIS ARTICLE describes and illustrates an interactive clinical model for communicating with children. The model is grounded in the kinds of relationships in which infants at risk can successfully engage and develop; it was developed in an interdisciplinary program for children with developmental disabilities. The focus was to establish parents, teachers, and other professionals as proactive partners in the child's social and communication development.

The fundamental thesis of the model is that children can learn to interact and communicate productively in each interpersonal contact. Further, it is proposed that attempts to foster social and communication development must not be limited to direct clinical and educational activities but must pervade the child's natural interactions. Another assumption is that a child's development in several domains (eg, cognitive, sensorimotor, communicative, emotional) is profoundly influenced by the styles of interaction that adults use with the child. Although the nativist view of development often prevails—for example, views such as "language just comes like hair and height"—there is increasing logical and empirical support for the view that language and other developmental competencies are in strong part a function of the quality and quantity of relationships in which the child evolves.[1-6] Several investigators of both developmental and emotional delays acknowledge that although biologic factors may play an initiating role in developmental problems, it is the caretaking environment that persists to impact the ultimate outcome.[7,8]

A third fundamental principle of the model is that children learn best by being more proactive than reactive. This occurs by children initiating contacts for learning and assuming the responsibility for creating their own learning reality in social contexts.[2,9] Widespread evidence from Piagetian-related studies demonstrates the active role a young child plays in his or her own natural learning.[10-12] Subsequently, other scholars and clinicians have extended Piaget's constructive view into the social realm where the issue is: How do children actively engage in order to become social and communicative? They propose that children become communicative to the degree to which they can act on and negotiate with their significant adults and peers. Consequently, in order for children to successfully communicate, they need to engage habitually with certain kinds of partners, ones whose styles allow the children to naturally learn to communicate and socially model from them.[2,3,13,14] This move to a social view of the child is further supported by a

Inf Young Children 1992; 4(3): 20–30

141

strong emerging movement known as *social constructivism*, which views a child as developing within socially embedded cultures (eg, parent-child, teacher-child, clinician-child).[10]

Regardless of their discipline, professionals' success with young children depends a great deal on their styles of communication; consequently it is proposed that several disciplines—education, parenting, physical therapy, psychology, physical education, nursing, pediatrics, and speech-language—consider the opportunity to fine-tune their communication with children as an opportunity to strengthen their own clinical and educational effects on the children. A more finely tuned communicative relationship with children can be expected to be beneficial for several reasons. First, children can learn to communicate and socialize in every interpersonal contact; thus every contact with a parent and professional is an opportunity for the child to learn either to communicate or not to do so.[14,15] Second, parents and professionals alike need children to be responsive and interactive with them in order to sustain themselves through the often difficult development of children with complications.[7,16] Third, the individual discipline's goals—whether refined motor, behavioral, cognitive, or health development or other—will be more readily reached if professionals communicate with children in ways that maintain the child's active engagement. Fourth, for many disciplines, communication is the primary vehicle for providing clinical or educational services; thus their effectiveness is keenly dependent on the nature of the communication relationship established. The partnership model is designed to facilitate the assessment, treatment, and parent education functions of several disciplines serving infants at risk. Recent laws (eg, Public Laws 94-142 and 99-457) have stimulated a revolution in early intervention that mandates parent involvement in the child's programming. The legislation specifies that all disciplines may be responsible for coordinating individual cases, and a critical aspect for coordinating cases is to clarify to parents and professionals how to most effectively communicate with the children. Finally, parents and families are becoming an increasing focus of services with infants, and communication is the universal tool families have to build relationships with children.

A series of studies of parents and teachers interacting with preconversational children at risk for developmental delays has revealed some relatively consistent patterns in the attitudes and beliefs of the adults, as well as in the interactive style of the children and adults.[3,13,17,18] What has been found repeatedly is a pattern of beliefs and communication styles that often run counter to an environment that would be expected to facilitate spontaneous communication development.

Parents involved in the partnership programs have revealed a perspective on language development that differs considerably from developmental findings on how communication develops in infancy. The parents' views also regularly minimized their own natural role in their child's learning to communicate. By and large, parents report that they are unsure as to what children need to do before they develop speech, and how they, the parents, can influence them. A paraphrase of their view on the source of language might be that "children grow into language much like they grow into clothes," with little need for help from parents. With such an attitude, parents often expected little active role for themselves in their child's language development. In the partnership programs,[3,17,19] clinicians educate parents in both their current and potential roles in their child's development. If parents and caregivers are unaware of the skills a child must have before language (eg, social play, turn taking, nonverbal communication, and purposeful play) they are unlikely to engage in productive relationships at the critical child developmental levels where communication is evolving.

Many parents and professionals appear to devalue their natural play and caregiving contacts as being critical to a child's communication. They often assume that if children are developmentally at risk, then only professional services provided directly to the child will help the child communicate.[3] They apparently do not appreciate the developmental influence that they are already providing the child on a daily basis in terms of their proactive but incidental interactions. Often adults fail to see that their daily interactions are naturally teaching the child to communicate; this process can be viewed as "natural therapy."[10] Once parents see the clear reciprocal effects they and their children have on each other, they become more respectful of their potential role and take an increasingly proactive role in their child's communication learning. A partnership model allows adults to capitalize on the natural successes they already have with the child.

A PROACTIVE PARTNERSHIP MODEL FOR INTERACTION

In response to the recurrent populations of children and adults with limited communicative relationships, a model of intervention has evolved from hundreds of individual parent-child communication programs and 20 years of interdisciplinary management of cases both in preschool classrooms and clinical teams. A system of clinical goals for both children and adults that is designed to strengthen natural communication relationships is shown in the box, "Goals To Facilitate Communication with Infants at Risk."

What follows is a partnership profile of adult and child interactions and beliefs that is a map of goals of the program, as well as a clinical profile professionals can use in addressing the question, "How can I build a more productive therapeutic relationship with infants at risk?" Research and clinical findings now converge on a number of generic styles of interaction that appear to provide the social support system for language to evolve.[2,3,7,13,18,20–22] In developing a partnership model, the investigators developed a clinical taxonomy of adult-child interaction styles that theory, research, and clinical studies agree are critical to a relationship for assisting communication development. The terms for the styles have been selected on the basis of their generic utility and the ease of consumer understanding.

Adult partnership styles for promoting social and communicative development

Following are two examples of an adult-infant interaction. They present contrasts in interactive styles that have been frequently observed in infants and adults across several diagnoses of risk. These examples will be referred to in the following discussion of adult styles.

Contrasting example

Early Sample

Jennifer: (Places a bowl of carrots and a spoon on the table near Jake while he watches.) "Okay, time to eat. How about some yummy carrots? You like carrots." (Picks child up from floor, puts in high chair.)
Jake: (Bangs spoon on high chair tray, smiles.)
Jennifer: "Are you (takes spoon) hungry after that nice, long nap?" (Raises spoon full of carrots to infant's mouth.) "Yum, yum. Open wide."
Jake: "Um." (opens mouth—leans toward mother.)
Jennifer: "Oh, you have such pretty teeth."

Later Sample

Jennifer: (Places bowl of carrots and spoon on the table near Jake while he watches; waits for a response from Jake.)
Jake: (Smiles, waves arms.) "Ah, ah."
Jennifer: (Outstretches arms toward Jake.) "Up."
Jake: (Raises arms up.) "Ah, ah."
Jennifer: (Puts child in high chair, holds up hands as if to ask "now what?")
Jake: (Bangs spoon on tray—smiles.)
Jennifer: "Hungry!" (Holds out hand for spoon—waits.)
Jake: (Waves spoon at mother—vocalizes gurgles.)
Jennifer: (Holds up spoon full of carrots.) "Yum, yum." (Waits expectantly.)
Jake: "Um." (Opens mouth—leans toward mother.)

Comments

The contrasting dialogues illustrate that both examples accomplish the same task results, but the child gets fewer opportunities to interact in the early example.

Goals To Facilitate Communication with Infants at Risk

Child goals

Social play
Increase interaction.
  Respond to others with interest.
  Prefer social contact to being alone.
  Enjoy being with people.

Turn taking
Stay in reciprocal interactions.
  Take turns with others.
  Share the lead in play.
  Imitate others' actions.
  Stay in give-and-take exchanges more than
    briefly.

Nonverbal communication
Establish an habitual nonverbal communica-
  tion with others before language.
  Communicate with movements and
    sounds.
  Communicate back and forth with others.
  Respond to others' speech.

Language
Express experiences and intentions in words
  and sentences for communication.
  Regularly say new words and combine
    words into sentences.
  Talk about own and other's interests and
    activities.

Conversation
Stay in balanced conversations for social rea-
  sons.
  Communicate for friendly contacts.
  Take turns in conversations.
  Keep conversation going.
  Stay on a topic more than momentarily.

Adult goals

Balance
Act and communicate as much as child does.
  Respond to child.
  Initiate contacts.
  Communicate for a response, then wait.
  Sustain joint activities.
Responsiveness
Sensitively and discriminatingly respond to
  emerging communication.
  Respond to child's interest and pace.
  Respond to child's actions as communica-
    tions.
  Respond to child's nonverbal communica-
    tion.

Match
Act and communicate in ways the child can
  do.
  Match actions, sounds, words.
  Show child how next to communicate.
  Be childlike.
Nondirectiveness
Follow the child's lead and allow him or her
  to share in the direction of the
    interaction.
  Follow child's lead.
  Comment more than using questions or
    commands.
  Limit questions to authentic ones.

Emotional attachment
Become spontaneously rewarding by
  engaging the child more for fun of it
    than to get something done.
  Actively enjoy child.
  Be animated.
  Show childlike play style.

Balancing

A first and influential adult style is balancing. This style of interaction refers to an adult and infant engaging in a give-and-take exchange together without one person assuming either a dominant or passive role. Each partner contributes about equally to the exchange. Often, the adult takes one action or communicative turn, then waits expectantly for the infant to take a turn. Each partner does about as much or says about as much as the other in his or her turn. Balanced exchanges can be described as *reciprocal*, in that each person influences the other. Reciprocity encourages the child to become actively involved in the interaction or communication, rather than take the passive, responsive role often characteristic of infants at risk and of developmentally delayed young children.[3,13,17,23,24]

Support for balanced adult-child relationships as crucial in early interactive and communicative development is apparent in theory and research,[25] language development,[2] emotional disorders,[7] parent-child relationship development,[14,26] and ecological views of development.[1,7] A basic notion supported by these theorists is that a child will learn from adults to the degree that the adult is a proactive partner who acts like the child, follows his or her motivations, and has a meaningful relationship in which give and take is the rule of interacting more than is a style of one-sided controls. Balanced relationships allow the infant to share the control of the direction and content of the interaction. Children appear to be more motivated to learn when they have some clear control over their environment and can exert significant effects on the adults close to them.[3,13,27]

Comments

In the first adult-infant example, Jennifer dominates the interaction by talking and acting much more than Jake does and controlling the direction of the exchange. Notice that even when Jake does try to send a message, Jennifer continues with her own agenda. By doing so, Jennifer is conveying to the boy that his actions and communications do not influence the environment.

Even activities like eating can involve balanced exchanges that assist a child in communicating. In the second example, Jennifer shares control of the activity with Jake, who clearly has effects on her. She also says and does about as much on her turn as Jake is capable of doing on his. Jake is not only more motivated to participate in eating, but he also actively participates in an interactive and communicative exchange as well.

How Can Adults Build Balanced Partnerships with Children?

In the partnership programs, parents and professionals use the following guide to monitor their interactive balance with infants:

- Occasionally, physically prompt the child to show how to initiate or take a turn.
- Wait expectantly for the child to initiate contact.
- Say or do one thing at the child's level; then wait.
- Give the child the time he or she needs to take his or her turn.
- Give the child some control in the interaction.
- Some of the time, keep the child for one more exchange.
- Share the choice of activities and topics with the child.
- Keep interactions going back and forth by responding in a meaningful way to his or her behaviors and communications.

Matching

Matching in adult-child interactions refers to the style with which a more developed person acts and communicates in ways the less developed person (often the infant or young child) can perform and in ways that relate meaningfully to the child's immediate experiences. By acting and communicating in ways similar to those used by the child, the adult provides feasible models for the child, thus increasing the likelihood that the child will succeed and stay for more interaction. A related strategy, known as *progressive matching*, refers to the adult communicating and interacting at an active and communicative level similar to that of the infant, while simultaneously showing the child a next developmental step. Matching is encouraged in at least three general ways. First, adults can match infants before they act or sound to increase the likelihood that they will interact and act more like the adult. Second, by matching after the infants' acts or sounds, adults encourage them to stay in the interaction for continued learning. Third, by generalized matching, the adults occasionally fine-tune their child's spontaneous behavior, regardless of whether it occurs in an interaction, to offer the child incidental learning opportunities.

The primary rationale for matching is that when an adult becomes finely tuned to a child's thoughts, communications, and interests, the adult models provided will be ones that the child will be motivated to spontaneously learn from within the interactions. Mahoney[13] has concluded that a child more easily learns actions, sounds, words, and ideas when they are ones the child can readily perform and when they do not exceed the child's current level of competence. When adults mismatch a child by performing far above the child's abilities or interests, the child often leaves the interaction and thus misses an opportunity to learn with the adult. Both cases limit infants from the frequent and sustained interactions they need to learn to communicate and become social partners.

The contrasting dialogue illustrates how an adult can shift from a relatively mismatched style to a more matched style that easily engages the child.

Comments

In the first example, Jennifer uses words to communicate, whereas Jake uses actions and sounds. Jennifer does not enter into Jake's world so that she can model his next step in communication; rather, she relies on words and sentences to convey her messages. Unfortunately, Jake remains in a world where all he sees or hears is too advanced to allow him to participate.

In the second example, the mother attracts Jake's attention by communicating in ways that he is able to, with sounds and gestures, and then frequently shows him a next way to communicate. In this example, Jake actively participates in the interaction and by the end seems to be developing a little conversational exchange, using actions and sounds similar to those used by his mother.

How Can Adults Build Matched Partnerships with Children?

The following list can be used by parents and professionals to monitor how they match their child:

- Respond to movements with similar movements and occasionally add a sound.
- Respond to sounds with similar sounds and occasionally a simple word like "hi," or a meaningful sound like "vrrroooom."
- Respond to a word with one or two words as if you were translating the child's meanings into your language and extending his or her ideas briefly.
- Respond to words with short phrases.
- Frequently act like the child in spontaneous contacts.
- Show the child a next developmental step by adding a sound, word, or communication to his or her turn.

Sensitive responsiveness

Although matching takes the adult into the child's world, it is also necessary for the adult to respond sensitively to the child in order to support his or her communication. Contingent responding across levels is also necessary; examples include responding to the child's primitive interactions,[27] his or her emerging nonverbal communication,[15,28] his or her conceptions and experiences,[29] his or her language and topic,[20] and his or her expressions of emotion.[7] Sensitive responding, then, is the active style that adults use to respond to their child's subtle developmental steps so that the child will pursue them also.

The value of sensitive adult responding is now becoming central to a wide variety of scholarly approaches to early education and child development.[12,13,30] One unifying feature of many recent approaches to social and communicative development is that learning proceeds best when it is focused on the child's current knowledge and experiences[2,14] rather than on adults' agenda or choices of goals. This growing respect for the child as being competent to best generate his or her own direction for learning encourages adults to take the role of a sensitive responder who is finely tuned to the child's current capacities and motivations.[22,31] Videotapes compiled for the research developing the partnership model, along with other recent research studies, show that the parents respond much less to their children's nonverbal behavior (that is, their actions and sounds) than to their verbal behavior.[3,32-34] This finding is cause for concern in light of developmental evidence that communication emerges from nonverbal behavior.[2,15] Adults who fail to respond to preverbal play, then, may be discouraging those subtle steps that develop into the child's social interactions and communications.

Comments

In the first exchange, the mother fails to respond to Jake's primitive communicative bids such as smiling and vocalizing. She plays a dominant role in this interaction, thereby placing Jake in a passive, responsive position. It should also be noted that Jake and his mother are participating in this exchange for different reasons. The mother wants only to complete feeding, whereas Jake appears interested in participating in a more social interaction .

The second dialogue illustrates a sensitively responsive mother who attends to Jake's actions and sounds as legitimate communications. She supports and encourages Jake's active participation in the exchange by responding to and interpreting his actions and sounds as meaningful.

How Can Adults Build Responsive Relationships with Children?

The following checklist can be used by adults to evaluate their own responsiveness:

- Respond to even the slightest behaviors or actions the child makes.
- Pay more attention to appropriate behaviors and less to immature or disruptive behaviors.
- Support and encourage the child's communications, even if they are less mature than communications made by his or her peers.
- Respond immediately to any behavior the child uses to initiate play.
- Adults can think of themselves as a "natural reinforcer" for the child. Be someone the child wants to play with so that he or she returns for more natural learning.

Child-based nondirectiveness

This partnership style follows the general rule that children learn more readily when they share the control and direction of interactions. The principle of nondirectiveness does not mean that all directions and controls are to be eliminated. However, social and communication development is more a matter of the child's self-motivated interactions than of behavior regulated by the adult.[35] Young children and infants at risk may not respond immediately to their parents or may be slow to respond. When this happens, many parents begin questioning and commanding, forcing the infant to leave his or her own interests and respond to their thoughts and motivations. Frequently, when a child placed in such a situation fails by not responding immediately, or correctly, or at all if unprompted, he or she may leave the interaction altogether.

On the other hand, a nondirective partnership style gives children the freedom to respond in the ways they are able and according to their own motivations and interests. Children will most likely experience some successes, which will encourage them to pursue future similar interactions. When adults assume a directive style of interaction, children experience frequent failure, thereby limiting their social contacts and reducing their opportunities to learn. When delayed infants or infants at risk primarily interact with controlling adults, their play style becomes passive; they may respond when directed but rarely pursue their own interests or abilities. Directing the child may also interfere with the natural learning of an activity. Children who are constantly directed and whose own motivations and interests are ignored may begin to believe that they are incompetent and that the right things to learn come from others' experiences and agenda rather than from their own.

Comments

In the first sample, Jennifer dominates the interaction by making repeated demands of Jake and imposing her agenda on the boy rather than following his lead. The mother's questions do not allow the child an opportunity to succeed. Jake has little opportunity to proactively participate in the contact, and he complies by playing a passive role that limits his opportunities to learn.

In the second sample, Jennifer demands and controls much less than in the first, and yet she gets much more actions and communications from Jake. As she follows his lead, she learns what is motivating him and is more successful building interactions on those motivations. Thus Jennifer gets her job of feeding accomplished, while at the same time providing considerable modeling and practice for communication development.

How Can Adults Build Nondirective Relationships With Children?

The following checklist can be used by various professionals to monitor their nondirectiveness in interactions:

- Limit questions and commands to authentic ones.
- Communicate by using comments, a powerful general strategy in motivating a child to communicate.

- Wait and expect: give the child time and signals to interact.
- Expect the child to communicate with the adult, at least some of the time.
- Match the child's language level and ideas.
- Build a habit of keeping the child for more than one turn.
- Allow the child to communicate from his or her interests and experiences much of the time, but also expect him or her to communicate about the adult's interests some of the time.

Emotional attachment

This partnership style embraces the idea that adults and infants achieve an emotional understanding of each other when their interactions are reciprocal and emotionally sensitive.[3,22] People can be emotional reinforcers for the child from early infancy on.[31] The child reacts to the appearance and disappearance of the adult and exerts considerable effort to maintain the adult's interaction. The presence of the infant's significant adult motivates the child to interact. In order for these interactions to become habitual and for emotional attachment to develop, mother and child each need to be effective in engaging the other.[27] However, infants at risk and children with delayed development may not experience the same rich, emotional attachments that normally developing children experience.[7] The stress and shock of giving birth to a delayed child may interfere with building the natural emotional partnership the child needs in order to pursue continued interactions.

The rationale for an emotional attachment between child and adult can be found in Goldberg's theory of social competence.[27] She predicted that when both the child and adult experience regular success with each other within habitual interactions, their emotional attachment will become deeper and stronger. When a child and adult feel competent together emotionally, they are combining their experiences of success with their actual cognitive and social achievements. Thus when adults experience greater success with their children (using the four previously discussed partnership principles to lead to successful feelings), there is a greater likelihood for increased emotional attachment. As emotional attachment increases, the likelihood that interactions will become habitual increases. Emotional attachment is important, not only in infancy, but at every stage of the child's development, in order for the child to more frequently pursue interactions and have the motivation to actively seek out social contacts with a variety of others throughout his or her life. Many parents of handicapped children appear to have an instrumental, instructive relationship with their child, rather than an animated, playful one.[13,23] This style appears to affect the extent to which the child may develop the kind of relationships that motivate him or her to become social and communicative.

Comments

In the first example, Jennifer is friendly and attentive to Jake, but she allows him little opportunity to express himself. Jake is unlikely to be emotionally invested in interactions that do not permit him to show what he knows and to have effects on others.

In the second example, Jake is having more effects on his mother and more opportunity to enjoy and express himself in an activity that was mainly task oriented in the first example. Here the mother and the boy each serve as spontaneous reinforcers for each other, with the emotional attachment providing a stronger motivation than the goal of the task.

How Can Adults Become Emotionally Attached to Children?

The emotional attachment between adult and child can be regularly monitored by a professional or parent in terms of the following issues:
- Ensure a genuine person-to-person contact.
- Balance turns with the child, focusing more on sustaining the interaction than getting a job done.
- Match the child's interests and communications.
- Respond sensitively to the child's emerging communications and behaviors that may become communications.
- Be nondirective; share the lead with the child, allowing him or her to communicate from his or her agenda and interests.
- Show the child that you are enjoying being with him or her.
- Actively reduce stress by focusing on play more than achievement.
- Avoid negative judgments or criticisms of the child.
- Concentrate on keeping the interaction going, rather than correcting his or her communication.
- Be more interesting than the child's distractions.

CONCLUSION

The challenge of building communicative relationships with infants at risk can have powerful preventive and therapeutic impacts for parents and professionals concerned with diverse developmental competencies. A partnership model of early intervention provides a consistent management approach for the various tasks faced by parents and professionals. At the Nisonger Center, several parents and professionals have adapted the partnership model to their own particular developmental focus with the child.

The recent legal mandates (PL 99-457) and the growing awareness of the value of the first months of life encourage an interdisciplinary focus on infants at risk and their families.[16,36-39] This article has proposed a model for communicating with infants and for supporting parent roles with the children. The model has been adapted to several common problems facing early intervention: motor development, emotional development, emergence of speech and language, and proactive parenting skills.

•   •   •

Professionals concerned with early intervention can prepare infants for the necessary prerequisite skills by integrating the five partnership styles into their daily interactions with children. An encapsulated profile of a partnership style of professional communication might be described as follows. By balancing, professionals not only provide children sufficient time and cues to initiate and respond, but also prepare them, early on, to not depend on others to interact and communicate for them when they may be capable of making attempts. By matching, professionals can teach parents and others that their children will communicate with them to the degree that the adults interact and communicate in ways the child can currently attempt. Thus professionals who are concerned about the child's language will move from a focus on developing sounds and words to a focus on finetuning themselves so that the child stays in the interaction for more spontaneous learning. The strategy of sensitive responding is critical for early communication, because it is here that adults recognize the power of their differential, attending more mature behaviors over less mature ones. Responding involves more than reacting to or answering the child; sensitive responding means taking the perspective of the child and reading his or her intentions and boundaries. By being nondirective, the language professional can show significant adults that infants will participate and practice more when adults follow the child's lead and avoid controlling the child according to the adults' agenda with constant questions and commands. Emotional attachment allows the adult to become a generalized motivator to the infant, a natural signal that is stress free and encourages successful engagements.

REFERENCES

1. Bronfenbrenner U. *The Ecology of Human Development.* Cambridge, Mass: Harvard University Press; 1979.
2. Bruner J. *Child Talk.* New York, NY: WW Norton; 1983.
3. MacDonald J. *Becoming Partners with Children: From Play to Conversation.* Chicago, Ill: Riverside Press, Inc; 1989.
4. Rosetti L. *High Risk Infants: Identification, Assessment, and Intervention.* Boston, Mass: College Hill Press; 1986.
5. Barnard KE, Bee HL. The assessment of parent–infant interaction by observation of feeding and teaching. In: Brazelton TB, Lester B, eds. *New Approaches to Developmental Screening in Infants.* New York, NY: Elsevier North Holland; 1989.

6. Farran DC, Kasari C, Yoder P, Harber L, Huntington GS, Comfort M. Rating mother-child inter-actions in handicapped and at-risk infants. In: Tamir, T, ed. *Stimulation and Intervention in Infant Development.* London, England: Freund Publishing House; 1987.

7. Greenspan S. *First Feelings: Milestones in the Emotional Development of Your Baby and Child.* New York, NY: Viking Penguin; 1985.

8. Meisels S, Shankoff N, eds. *Early Intervention. A Handbook of Theory, Practice, and Analysis.* New York, NY: Cambridge University Press; 1989.

9. Vygotsky LS. *Mind in Society.* Cambridge, Mass: Harvard University Press.

10. Kegan R. *The Evolving Self: Continuous Development of Meaning.* Cambridge, Mass: Harvard University Press; 1981.

11. Piaget J. *The Origins of Intelligence in Children.* New York, NY: Norton; 1952.

12. Rosenberg S, Robinson C. Enhancement of mother's interactional skills in an infant education program. *Education Training Mentally Retarded.* 1985;163–169.

13. Mahoney G. Enhancing the developmental competence of handicapped infants. In: Marfo K, ed. *Parent-Child Interaction and Developmental Disabilities.* New York, NY: Praeger; 1988.

14. Stern D. *The Interpersonal World of the Infant. A View From Psychoanalysis and Developmental Psychology.* New York, NY: Basic Books; 1985.

15. Bates E. *Language and Context: The Acquisition of Pragmatics.* New York, NY: Academic Press; 1976.

16. Gallagher JJ, Beckman P, Cross AH. Families of handicapped children: Sources of stress and its amelioration. *Except Child.* 1983;50:10–19.

17. Gillette Y. *Ecological Programs for Communicating Partnerships: Models and Cases.* Chicago, Ill: Riverside Press, Inc; 1989.

18. MacDonald J, Carroll J. A social partnership model for assessing early communication develop-ment. *Lang Speech Hearing Schools.* In press.

19. Gillette Y, MacDonald J. *ECO Resources.* Chicago, Ill: Riverside Press, Inc; 1989.

20. Cross TG. Habilitating the language impaired child: Ideas from parent-child interaction. *Top Lang Dis.* 1985;4:1–4.

21. Nelson K. *Narratives from the Crib.* Cambridge, Mass: Harvard University Press; 1989.

22. Trevarthan LB. Communication and cooperation in early infancy: A description of primary intersubjectivity. In: Bullowa M, ed. *Before Speech: The Beginnings of Communication.* London, England: Cambridge University Press; 1979.

23. Girolometto L. Developing dialogue skills: The effects of a conversational model of language intervention. In: Marfo K, ed. *Parent-Child Interaction and Developmental Disabilities: Theory, Research, and Intervention.* New York, NY: Praeger; 1988.

24. Tannock R. Control and reciprocity in mothers' interactions with Down's Syndrome and normal children. In: Marfo K, ed. *Parent-Child Interaction and Developmental Disabilities: Theory, Re-search, and Intervention.* New York, NY: Praeger; 1988.

25. Marfo K, ed. *Parent-Child Interaction and Developmental Disabilities: Theory, Research, and Intervention.* New York, NY: Praeger; 1988.

26. Kaye K. *The Mental and Social Life of Babies: How Parents Create Persons.* Chicago, Ill: Univer-sity of Chicago Press; 1982.

27. Goldberg S. Social competence in infancy: A model of parent-infant interaction. *Merril-Palmer Q.* 1977; 23:263–277.

28. Sugarman S. The development of preverbal communications: Its contribution and limits in promoting the development of language. In: Schiefelbusch R, Pickar J, eds. *The Acquisition of Communicative Competence.* Baltimore, Md: University Park Press; 1984.

29. Snow C. Parent-child in teaching and the development of communicative ability. In: Schiefelbusch R, Pickar J, eds. *The Acquisition of Communicative Competence.* Baltimore, Md: University Park Press; 1984.

30. Elkind D. *Miseducation: Preschools at Risk.* New York, NY: Knopf; 1987.

31. Newsom J. The growth of shared understanding between infant and caregiver. In: Bullowa M, ed. *Before Speech: Interpersonal Communications.* London, England: Cambridge University Press; 1979.

32. Erheart B. Mother-child interactions with nonretarded and mentally retarded preschoolers. *Am J Ment Defic.* 1982;87:20–25.

33. Jones OH. Prelinguistic communication skills in Down's Syndrome and normal infants. In: Field TM, Goldberg S, Stern D, Sostek AM, eds. *High Risk Infants and Children: Adults and Peer Interactions.* New York, NY: Academic Press; 1980.

34. Peterson G, Sherrod K. Relationship of maternal language to language development and language delay in children. *Am J Ment Defic.* 1982;86:503–511.

35. Deci E. *Intrinsic Motivation.* New York, NY: Plenum Press; 1975.

36. Bailey D, Simeonsson R, eds. *Family Assessment in Early Intervention.* Columbus, Ohio: Merrill Publishing Co; 1988.

37. Fewell RR. Assessing handicapped infants. In: Garwood SG, Fewell RR, eds. *Educating Handicapped Infants.* Rockville, Md: Aspen; 1983.

38. Bullova M. *Before Speech: The Beginnings of Interpersonal Communication.* London, England: Cambridge University Press; 1979.

39. Affleck G, McGrade BJ, McQueeney M, Allen D. Promise of relationship-focused early intervention in developmental disabilities. *J Spec Educ.* 1982;16: 413–430.

A relationship-based approach to self-reliance in young children with motor impairments

Robert S. Marvin, PhD
Assistant Professor
Department of Pediatrics

Robert C. Pianta, PhD
Associate Professor
Curry School of Education
University of Virginia
Charlottesville, Virginia

THERE ARE OFTEN wide differences in quality of life among children and families despite similarities in the severity of the children's disabilities. Although the early literature on families of children with disabilities tended to discuss differences between these families and families of nondisabled children as reflecting dysfunction,[1] recent studies suggest that the differences between "normal" and "handicapped" families may represent distinct but equally workable adaptations to different conditions faced by each type of family.[2]

In the Child-Parent Attachment Project at the University of Virginia's Kluge Children's Rehabilitation Center and Research Institute, we are studying how families adapt to having a child with a developmental disability. Through the use of a number of standardized, videotaped interactive measures and interviews in a homelike laboratory environment, we are collecting extensive data on families who have young children (18 to 48 months) with cerebral palsy (CP).

Three basic ideas serve as the foundation for this project. The first is that many quality of life outcomes (eg, self-reliance) start early in life. The second is that, within the group of children with CP, differences in self-reliance are as much related to a child's relationships with family members as they are to differences in specifics of the child's physical disability. The third is that attachment theory and the procedures used in attachment research[3-6] may provide powerful tools for studying individual differences in quality of life outcomes.

In this article we present (1) some lessons gained from research in normal development that are important guidelines for thinking about children with physical disabilities, (2) concepts from attachment theory and research that are applicable to this topic, (3) two case studies of preschool children with CP to illustrate the link between self-reliance and the quality of the child's attachment to his mother, and (4) differences in the mothers' thoughts and feelings about their relationships both with their children and with their own parents that may account for differences in the self-reliance of their children. (To avoid confusion and awkward

---

Supported by NIH grant R01 HD 26911. An earlier version of this article was presented at the annual meeting of the National Center for Clinical Infant Programs, Washington, DC, December 7, 1991. The authors acknowledge the assistance of Leigh Berry, MA, Gretchen Lovett, Christina Lopez, MA, Thomas O'Conner, Karen Rogers, MA, and Stacey Watkins, MA.

Inf Young Children 1992; 4(4): 33–45

sentence construction, we use the female pronoun to refer to the adult attachment figure and the masculine pronoun to refer to the individual [child or adult] who is attached to that figure.)

LESSONS FROM THE STUDY OF NORMAL DEVELOPMENT

Recently there has been increased emphasis on studying, and intervening with, high-risk children by using the same theories and procedures employed in the study of normal development processes.[7] In this section we discuss four lessons from the study of normally developing children that have implications for our work with children with motor impairments.

Developmental pathways for quality of life outcomes start in infancy and early childhood

Much developmental research indicates that the period of infancy and early childhood lays the foundation for later quality of life outcomes. Competence in certain domains (eg, self-reliance) in infancy predicts competence in similar domains in adolescence and early adulthood.[8] This does not mean that later outcomes are fixed in infancy or that there is no room for intervention in the interim. The developmental approach we advocate is therefore a preventive perspective. Our goal is to identify risk early in development, during periods in which successful interventions may have the short- and long-term result of altering the course of development toward a more functional pathway.

Developmental pathways involve the child's relationships with caregivers

There is a growing literature on normal and high-risk children that indicates that child outcomes such as self-reliance, personal competence, and rewarding interpersonal relationships (assessed as late as adolescence and young adulthood) have roots in the child's experiences with caregivers in infancy and early childhood.[9] The pathways for development of quality of life outcomes are chosen, in large part, by the quality of the relationships that the infant and young child experiences with caregivers.[10] The approach we take to studying these early relationships is based on attachment theory.

Alternative pathways exist for attaining quality of life outcomes

It is clear from many studies of children's social, cognitive, and language development that, despite wide-ranging capacities in these domains, most children develop adequate self-reliance, personal competence, and rewarding interpersonal relationships; for the majority of the population, competent development is the rule. This suggests that there are alternative developmental pathways toward the same or similar outcome(s).

This notion of alternative developmental pathways is particularly important for the study of children with developmental disabilities. Because they experience impairments in one or more basic sensory, information-processing, or motor systems (eg, locomotion or sight), their development may not follow the same pathway as that of a nonimpaired child. Yet most clinicians know, and base much of their work on the fact, that children with disabilities can and often do attain many of the same outcomes as normally developing children.

The most visible example of alternate pathways is the use of mechanical and/or electronic prosthetics for children with sensory or motor impairments (eg, orthotics, motorized wheelchairs, and electronic communication boards). These prosthetics offer an alternative pathway to the same functional outcome. Less visible but equally important are accommodations made in the caregiver–child relationship that offer these alternative pathways. For example, we have shown that some nonlocomotor children with CP have a secure attachment with their primary caregiver despite the fact that the locomotor system is, in normal children, of primary importance in developing that secure relationship. In those dyads with secure, nonlocomotor children, the caregiver adopts certain practices that function as a prosthetic in that crucial developmental area, again facilitating an alternative pathway to the same outcome.[11] Other studies of children with disabilities have suggested that similar, alternative strategies take place at the level of family organization.[2]

Individual skill-based and relationship-based approaches

Assessment and intervention with infants and young children are usually aimed at documenting the presence or absence of certain skills or behaviors and then training the child to acquire the missing skills. This skill focus, however, is only part of the landscape we need to see to enhance effectively the quality of life for these children. In real-life development these behaviors do not occur in a vacuum. They have a behavioral context and function; that is, they accomplish something meaningful for the child. For example, visual motor skills such as orienting, grasping, and locomotion serve such developmental functions as pleasurable exploration of the physical environment, intentional movement from point A to point B, and organization of physical proximity and contact between the child and his attachment figure.

Oftentimes, in traditional efforts to assess and intervene at the level of individual child skills and behaviors, we pay little attention to these functions. In some ways, this is a forest and trees problem; we may be successful in training a child to grasp objects or crawl, but in our efforts to do so we may miss the fact that the child is not using those, or other, behaviors functionally to explore pleasurably the physical environment. Moreover, in our efforts to assess and train individual behaviors and skills, we may not attend to the alternative pathways through which the child might more easily accomplish the function served by the skills we are working so hard to train.

We propose that developmental functions such as self-reliance are actually accomplished in normally developing children as well as in children with disabilities at the dyadic or relationship level. Interestingly, this is often because the caregiver acts as a type of prosthetic, even for the nonimpaired child. Although we do not advocate abandoning skill-based approaches, we do propose that individual child behaviors and skills are perhaps less important in determining whether some outcome or function will be achieved than the quality of the child–caregiver interaction. In the next section we review a research paradigm that provides an empiric framework for this approach.

ATTACHMENT THEORY AND RESEARCH

Development of attachment

As developed by Bowlby,[4] Ainsworth et al,[3] and others, attachment theory proposes that infants are born with, or develop relatively soon after birth, a number of attachment behaviors such as crying, sucking, smiling, visual tracking, and, later, following and clinging that predictably elicit adult caregiving behaviors. Over the course of the first 6 to 9 months of life, stable patterns of interaction become established between parents and infant such that when the infant is hungry, frightened, or otherwise distressed physical proximity and contact between the caregiver and infant are the predictable outcome, and the infant is soothed, comforted, and/or cared for. Attachment behaviors, and the accompanying patterns of parent-infant interaction, are highly regulated by the dyad and serve the evolutionary function of protecting the infant from danger during the period in which he is developing the skills necessary to protect himself and to become integrated in a self-reliant way within a larger social network.

Toward the end of the first year of life a number of profound changes take place in the organization of the infant's attachment behavior system. These changes are due in part to new developmental skills in the infant's repertoire. Among these are the onset of locomotion, object and person permanency, the ability to construct a plan for gaining or maintaining proximity to and/or contact with the attachment figure, and the ability to assess his attachment figure's availability to him and in simple ways to anticipate her behavior.

With these new abilities, the infant is now able to use his attachment figure as a secure base for exploration.[3,12] This concept refers to the infant's tendency to move away from the mother to explore as long as he feels that he can get back to her if he wishes. What tends to happen is that the infant or young child assesses his ability to gain proximity to his attachment figure, and if he feels secure that he will be able to do so he moves off to explore, perhaps occasionally returning to her briefly to refuel before moving off again. If he is frightened or distressed, however, or if the attachment figure leaves or behaves in some unpredictable way, the infant immediately stops exploring and seeks proximity or contact with her. Once contact is achieved, the infant (if necessary) is soothed, and if he again perceives the attachment figure as stationary or at least easily accessible the balance tips back in favor of exploration, and he again moves off. In a critical way, the developmental milestone of exploration from a secure base is a milestone achieved by the dyad, not merely by the infant.

Working models

Bowlby,[4,13] Bretherton,[14] Main et al,[15] and others have proposed that the infant internalizes the interactions between his caregivers and himself in the form of internal working models of those caregivers and of the self. These are what allow him to appraise the situation in which he finds himself, to anticipate his caregiver's behavior, to assess various alternatives for his own action, to choose among those alternatives, and to carry out a planned course of behavior. Internal working model refers to many of the same internal processes that traditionally have been referred to as cognitive or social-cognitive activities.

These models are, of course, relatively primitive in infancy and become progressively more sophisticated and differentiated as the child develops. Even in an infant 10 to 12 months of age, however, these models represent typical patterns of interaction that the infant has had with his caregivers, his own ideas of what behaviors he has available to himself to cope with his world, and likelihoods about his caregiver's behavior (eg, whether or not she is likely to respond to his bid for physical contact).

Individual differences in attachment

Internal working models develop out of, and in turn influence, individual differences in patterns of infant–parent interaction.[3] The relationship-based model we propose explicitly endorses the child's contribution to these individual differences (eg, temperament, intelligence quotient, and constraints of specific medical complications). Space limitations do not allow discussion of these complex issues, however. The great bulk of research on individual differences in attachment has relied on the "strange situation," a 20-minute procedure developed by Ainsworth et al[3] for use with their Baltimore sample. This videotaped, standardized, laboratory procedure involves a free play episode with both mother and infant in the room and the subsequent introduction of a friendly stranger. In turn, this is followed by two separations and reunions between infant and mother. Detailed analysis of the videotape leads to classification of the infant into one of the following three major categories.

1. *Secure (group B)*. This child's attachment figure is usually sensitive and responsive to his attachment behavior. He will tend to use her as a secure base for exploration. In the strange situation he will approach her easily if distressed and will be easily comforted. Most studies suggest that about 65% to 70% of children fall into this group.

2. *Insecure-avoidant (group A)*. This child's attachment figure tends to ignore or reject his attachment behavior. He will be less likely to use her as a secure base for exploration, having a tendency to go it on his own and thus to place himself at some risk. In the strange situation he will be less distressed by separation and will tend to avoid his mother on reunion. The data suggest that approximately 20% of children fall into this group.

3. *Insecure-resistant (group C)*. This child's attachment figure tends to be unpredictable, insensitive, and sometimes intrusive in responding to his attachment behavior. This child will be least likely to use her as a secure base for exploration. In the strange situation he will tend not to explore, become extremely distressed on separation from her, and on reunion react with an ambivalent or passive combination of wanting contact with her while at the same time rejecting that contact. Approximately 10% to 15% of children are in this group.

Each of these categories reflects a coherent strategy on the infant's part for coping with the friendly stranger and with the mother's departures and returns. More recently, Main and Soloman[16,17] have identified a fourth group of children who appear to have no coherent strategy for coping with the separations and reunions. These infants appear to be disoriented, disorganized, and even fearful toward the mother.

Main and Soloman[16,17] have labeled these infants *insecure-disorganized (group D)*. In many situations involving attachment-caregiving interactions, this caregiver tends to behave in frightened or frightening ways. She tends not to function as a stable, competent caregiver of at least the child's emotional needs, and the child is generally not able to use her as a secure base for exploration. In the strange situation this child will tend to respond to separation and reunion with behavior patterns that appear contradictory or disorganized (eg, being distressed during separation but then remaining completely motionless when the attachment figure returns). It is uncertain at this time what percentage of children fall into this group: The percentage varies depending on the degree of psychosocial, and perhaps medical, risk.

The reader is referred to Ainsworth et al,[3] Cassidy and Marvin,[18] and Main and Soloman[17] for details of the strange situation procedure, details about classifying infants into the four groups, and descriptions of the behavior patterns typical of each group.

Quality of attachment and other childhood outcomes

Over the past 20 years a large body of research has demonstrated that the quality of a child's attachment to his caregiver(s) is closely related to both concurrent and future outcomes. From their original Baltimore study, Ainsworth and colleagues[3] found that securely attached infants were more competent during the last quarter of the first year of life in a number of areas, including a smoother balance in use of the mother as a secure base for exploration, the development of object and person permanency, and cooperation/compliance with the mother's instructions and admonitions. In their large Minnesota project, Erickson and colleagues[19] found that attachment at 1 year of age predicts a number of child outcomes well into the elementary school years, including social competence with peers, compliance with parents and teachers, self-control, and self-esteem. A number of ongoing projects are continuing to find strong relationships between the quality of a child's attachment(s) and other personal and social competencies in normal and at-risk samples.[20-22] It is consistent with our focus on the importance of relationships that the strongest measures in all these studies tend to reflect interactions between the child and others rather than individual characteristics of the child himself.

Stability of attachment into adulthood and parenthood

Recently, George and colleagues[23] and Main and Goldwyn[24] have developed a procedure for assessing the quality of an adult's working models, or internal representations, regarding his relationships with his own attachment figure(s). In an approximately 1-hour interview called the Adult Attachment Interview (AAI), the individual is asked a series of questions designed to elicit detailed memories about childhood attachment experiences, thoughts about the effects of those experiences on his adult personality, and thoughts about the importance of intimate relationships. Analysis of both the content and the quality of the responses provides a classification of the individual's current state of mind with respect to attachments as either autonomous, dismissing, preoccupied, or unresolved. The basic differences among these groups are briefly outlined below.

Autonomous. The autonomous individual is coherent, believable, and objective in discussing his early attachment experiences; has easy access to relevant memories; clearly values close relationships; and feels comfortable depending on others.

He may or may not have a difficult early attachment history, but if so he has managed to grow beyond it and is now comfortable in close relationships.

Dismissing. This individual dismisses the importance of attachments and of the emotions associated with them. Currently, he tends to speak easily of early negative experiences but dismisses their effect on himself as an adult, or he tends to discuss attachments at an abstract level that is clearly separated from related emotions. He may steadfastly insist that he has no memory of attachment experiences in his early childhood, or he may idealize his attachment figures without being able to gain access to specific memories that support his statements.

Preoccupied. This individual is confused and preoccupied about his relationship(s) with his own attachment figure(s). He remains unable to move beyond this enmeshed relationship, either unsuccessfully struggling with it in an angry and conflicted way or accepting it in a passive and vague way.

Unresolved. During the AAI, individuals sometimes report the loss of an important attachment figure or the experience of abuse or some other disorganizing trauma. Many of these individuals go on to report a successful process of grieving over or mourning this loss or trauma and of having reorganized their lives and moved on. Others, however, respond to the questions in a manner indicating that they currently remain unresolved. Their responses include at least some of the following: unusually strong bereavement behaviors; continuing excessive fear, guilt, or worry about the relationship; lack of ability to discuss the loss or trauma; feelings of having caused the trauma themselves; or excessive general confusion about the trauma. Overall, their responses indicate that they remain disorganized by the trauma, and they may speak of it as if the crisis of the trauma continues in full force in the present, even though it may have happened years ago.

There is increasing evidence that an adult's classification on the AAI corresponds to his child's behavior toward him in the strange situation. For example, in retrospective studies Main and Goldwyn[24] and Grossman et al[25] report high concordance coefficients between mother and child attachment classification. Fonagy et al[26] report 75% concordance between the AAI classifications of women during the last trimester of their first pregnancy and their infants' classification in the strange situation 1 year after the birth.

In summary, evidence suggests that distinct, stable patterns emerge early in this relationship, have a significant influence on personal and interpersonal competence through childhood and adulthood, and even tend to be passed on to the succeeding generation.

ATTACHMENT AND SELF-RELIANCE IN CHILDREN WITH CEREBRAL PALSY: TWO CASE STUDIES

In the previous sections we presented the case for taking a relationship-based approach to the study of children with developmental disabilities and then reviewed the research on child–parent attachment as a potentially powerful model for implementing that approach. We now return to our original problem and re-state that problem in terms of three specific questions, which are framed in attach-ment/relationship terms:

1. Can we see these differential patterns of self-reliance and overdependence in young children with CP?
2. Are these patterns related to the quality of the child's attachment to his primary caregiver?
3. Are these patterns further related to the primary caregivers' working mod-els of their relationships both with their children and with their own attach-ment figures?

Procedures

We present two case studies from our project. The two children were approxi-mately 3 1/2 years old and were from comparable families as measured by a number of demographic variables.

Strange situation. Each of the children participated in a modified version of the strange situation adapted for children who are nonlocomotor.[11]

Self-reliance task. The mother sits on the floor, supporting or holding her child in front of her as necessary. The child is shown a battery-powered toy operated by a switch pad. The mother is instructed that we would like her child to play with the toy and that she can help him when and to the extent to which she thinks that help is needed. In a series of steps, the task becomes increasingly difficult because of the progressive addition of extra, widely spaced switch pads required to operate the toy. The procedure is videotaped and scored from the tape. The scoring proce-dure is based on our conceptualization that self-reliance is a relationship-based construct reflecting an individual's working model of himself as one who can en-joy tackling a difficult task and who can easily, and trustingly, ask for help when he requires it.

Child 1

Strange situation. The mother sat on the floor, supporting her child on her lap while the child explored. Throughout this episode the mother watched the child's activity closely and took her cues to help from his behavior (ie, she was sensitive to what he was trying to do at any moment, gave him help promptly but only when he needed it, and organized her help so that it consisted of the minimum necessary for the child to succeed in what he was trying to do). The mother and child re-mained happy and focused on exploration. When the stranger joined them, the child interacted with her in further exploring the toys.

When the mother left the room, the child cried hard immediately. The stranger eventually succeeded in calming the child, and he returned to playing but only halfheartedly.

When the mother reentered the room and greeted him, the child turned toward her, smiled broadly, and became quite excited and animated. As she approached him, he reached for her, looked directly at her, and vocalized happily. The mother picked him up, and they returned to exploration with the same focus and enjoyment as during the first episode. This overall pattern of behavior is consistent with a classification of securely attached.

Self-reliance task. The child enjoyed the toy and remained completely focused on it. As the task became more complex, he was unable to operate it. Each time he failed, he looked either at the experimenter, mother, or father with a smile. The mother helped him promptly, providing him only with the minimal amount of physical help necessary for him to succeed on each step of the procedure.

This pattern is consistent with a classification of self-reliant. Most important, the dyad accomplished much more than would be suggested by the severity of the child's motor impairment.

Child 2

Strange situation. This dyad began in much the same fashion as the first, with the mother supporting the child while he explored. This child, however, did not remain focused on playing with the toys; he asked questions about the whereabouts of his brother. When the stranger entered, he interacted easily with her.

When the mother got up to leave, the child was sitting independently on the floor. As the mother walked out of the room, he called her and then immediately broke into loud screaming and threw himself back on the floor in an almost violent fashion. He vigorously rejected the stranger's attempts to console him, and again threw himself backward when she raised him into a sitting position. At that point, as is standard practice, we asked the mother to return to the room early.

The child continued crying after the mother entered the room and picked him up. After approximately 15 seconds, the crying diminished to strong fussing, and he angrily and repeatedly told his mother he would not play. It took the mother a full 3 minutes to calm him, and even then he returned to playing without much focus and with some helpless whining.

This pattern of behavior is consistent with a classification of insecure with a combination of the insecure-resistant and insecure-disorganized categories. This child never did use his mother as a secure base for focused exploration.

Self-reliance task. This child easily operated the toy with only one switch. As the number of switches was increased, however, he behaved in an increasingly helpless way. The mother repeatedly tried to get him to think of what he needed to do to operate the toy, but the child paid little attention to what she was saying. He began asking for help in a whining tone and eventually began crying in an angry tone. Although it seemed extremely important to the mother that her child succeed on the task, she never did physically help him operate the toy, and given his level of physical capability this dyad successfully completed surprisingly few steps of the procedure.

This pattern is much less consistent with a classification of self-reliant; rather, the child behaved in a helpless and dependent/angry manner.

CHILD ATTACHMENT AND PARENTAL WORKING MODELS OF CLOSE RELATIONSHIPS

As we continue to collect data, we are seeing with great frequency the pattern outlined above, in which a secure attachment is associated with self-reliance and an insecure attachment with an angry and overdependent lack of self-reliance. The question now arises as to what factors may account for the distinctly different developmental pathways taken by each of these children and the relationships of which they are a part. Our first approach to answering this question was to examine what might be called ecologic factors in the caregiving environment. The second was to examine maternal factors that might affect the mother's caregiving behavior.

Ecologic factors in the caregiving environment

Each mother was interviewed, and completed standardized questionnaires, about seven ecologic factors: social support, marital satisfaction, family distribution of caregiving tasks, financial contributions, out-of-home day care, leisure time, and organized family daily routines. The only difference between these two families on any of these measures was that family 1 placed their child in day care for 25 hours per week whereas family 2 did so for 40 hours per week. In both cases, the maternal grandmother was the day-care provider.

Thus it appears that these ecologic factors do not distinguish between the families and would not account adequately for the differences between the children. In fact, to avoid any misperceptions we should clearly state that both these families are seen by their clinic staff, and by others, as well organized, highly functioning families. We turn now to maternal factors.

Maternal working models

We present excerpts from and discuss three separate interviews administered to each of these mothers: the Parent Development Interview, the Reaction of the Diagnosis Interview, and the AAI.

Parent Development Interview

The first interview is a variation of the Parent Development Interview.[27] It consists of 20 questions that elicit details about the mother's thoughts and feelings in parenting this child as well as specific memories of those experiences. An open, balanced, and secure working model of parenting is characterized by thoughtful, noncontradictory perceptions of the child and the relationship. Responses to the questions suggest that the mother is sensitive to her child's needs and signals. She comfortably accepts the child as he is. She also has easy access to specific positive and negative memories and feelings involved in parenting this child.

A defended or dismissing working model of parenting is characterized by lack of memory for feelings and/or events. The mother may idealize the child and the relationship without being able to provide specifics that back up her statements and make them believable.

An enmeshed, preoccupied working model of parenting is again characterized by much confusion and/or distress. The individual is preoccupied with the child and his problems while at the same time meaning and to be sensitive to the child's signals. These parents communicate a lack of comfortable acceptance of the child as he is.

Mother 1. The mother began the interview by describing specific aspects of her relationship with her son in a calm, thoughtful, and even joyful way. The interview then continued:

> *Interviewer:* Do you ever feel really needy as a parent?
>
> *Mother* (after a thoughrful moment): Yes, sometimes . . . when it gets to be so much . . . almost more than you can take. Sometimes you wonder why it had to happen to you.
>
> *Interviewer:* All parents struggle with knowing how much to push their child to do what is difficult versus how much not to push. What kinds of situations do you struggle with in this area?
>
> *Mother:* Well, I guess I do struggle with that. I don't want to make him do something he just can't do . . . but he can do a lot. You encourage him to do everything he can . . . I think he'll gain a lot more that way . . . I feel like he'll let us know when he's had enough.

This mother presented an open, balanced working model of parenting. She was thoughtful and concise and had easy access to both feelings and memories. She was sensitive toward and accepting of her child while being aware of the dilemmas she faces as a parent.

Mother 2. This mother began the interview by describing her relationship with her son as loving, caring, and interesting. Despite a long and rambling response, she was unable to describe an incident that illustrated loving.

> *Interviewer:* Can you give me a specific memory that illustrates how your relationship is "caring?"

> *Mother:* Well, I think the term *cerebral palsy* makes everybody think you just got to take care of him all the time . . . I don't know why, but that's what people seem to think.

> *Interviewer:* Do you ever feel really needy as a parent?

> *Mother* (after immediately beginning to cry): Hmmmm . . . not really, no . . . because I've determined that we're going to make an effort to help him out, and there aren't going to be any obstacles in the way . . . if there are, we'll just go over them.

> *Interviewer:* All parents struggle with knowing how much to push their child to do what is difficult versus how much not to push. What kinds of situations bring up this dilemma for you?

> *Mother* (with a determined look on her face): With him, you've got to push him every minute of every day, you've got to push.

The mother then started to cry again and went into a long and confusing statement about her distress over the fact that others sometimes feel she pushes too hard.

This mother's working model of her relationship with her son is enmeshed/ preoccupied. Throughout the interview she answered questions about her son by referring more to herself than to him. She did not have easy access to specific memories of events in their relationship, and many of her answers were rambling and confusing. She cried throughout most of the interview and communicated many conflicting feelings without communicating any awareness of them. She actively denied any feelings of neediness, anger, guilt, or pain in their relationship. Finally, she seemed not to accept her child as he is but rather seemed to take on the CP as a mission.

Reaction to Diagnosis Interview

This is an interview developed in our laboratory to study parents' reactions to their children's diagnosis and the degree to which they have resolved the grief and crisis of that diagnosis. It consists of 10 questions that cover feelings and specific experiences regarding the initial realization that the child had a problem, the process of diagnosis, ideas about why this happened to them, and how the thoughts and feelings have changed over the time since the diagnosis.

Parents classified as resolved communicate, with concrete memories, that they have gone through the grief process. More important, they communicate through words and affect that the crisis and the intense feelings are now in the past.

Parents who are unresolved tend not to have grieved openly, or only in a limited way. Although they may state that they have accepted the diagnosis, either their affect during the interview or the content of their responses suggests otherwise. Typically these parents either evade direct discussion of relevant experiences and feelings or seem grief-stricken during the interview and seem to have taken on the mission of overcoming the diagnosis. Many communicate openly that the feelings at the time of the diagnosis continue unabated.

Mother 1. This mother began the interview by communicating clear memories of the period of time over which she came to realize that there was something wrong with her child. She leaned forward and looked the interviewer in the eyes while she was talking but remained calm. The interview continued:

> *Interviewer:* What were your feelings at the time you received the diagnosis?
>
> *Mother:* Well . . . it wasn't very nice . . . it was kind of hard, you know, to think that our child had CP . . . you know, we didn't know what it was all about or what was going to happen.
>
> *Interviewer:* How have these feelings changed over time? Mother (after a thoughtful pause): Well . . . you learn to accept it . . . you learn to live with it. There's still times we think . . . we wonder if he were a normal 3-year-old, what he could do, what you wouldn't have to do . . . for the most part, that's just [child's name] . . . it's more of an accepted thing that that's the way he is.

This mother was classified as resolved because of her calm affect, her thoughtful ability to gain access to memories and feelings about the period of diagnosis, and her clear indication that she has placed this period in the past without forgetting it. She was also able to communicate continuing thoughts about what might have been without becoming preoccupied and absorbed in feelings of grief.

Mother 2. This mother presented a long narrative of the sequence of events leading to the diagnosis, including much focus on how individuals within the health care system were insensitive to her needs and distress at that time. She continued to cry during most of this narrative.

> *Mother* (continuing to cry and attempting to regain control): I'm sorry for all this crying.
>
> *Interviewer:* That's OK . . . remember you said it's still an "open wound."

Mother: Yes, and it probably always will be. And you'd think that four years later at least it would diminish!

Interviewer: You haven't found that it's diminished?

Mother (continuing to cry): No . . . in fact I think it's even stronger!

Although this mother's story tends to evoke appropriate sympathy, it is clear that she is unresolved with respect to the diagnosis. She seems unable to move past the crisis period and in fact feels that it is getting worse.

Research questions

We can now return again to our original questions. Within the limitations of a two-case study procedure, we have some compelling suggestions regarding the origins of the differences between the two children discussed above. Specifically we suggest that, having resolved the crisis of the diagnosis, the first mother is in a freer, more autonomous position to perceive and respond sensitively to her child's signals and needs. The second mother's lack of resolution of the diagnosis, and her preoccupation with her own pain and distress, could certainly interfere with her ability to be as sensitive.

One question still remains. Given the other similarities between these mothers, what could account for the difference in how each has managed to deal with the diagnosis? Stemming from the work of Main and others, our hypothesis is that differences in each mother's working models regarding her own attachment figures might be one important factor.

Adult Attachment Interview

Mother 1. This mother described her early relationship with her mother as happy, sad, and recently more loving. She described her relationship with her father as angry and more recently as forgiving. She went on to describe experiences of physical abuse from her father toward her mother and siblings. When she was upset as a young child she seemed to go off by herself rather than to her mother. Sometime during the intervening years, however, she had thoughtfully reevaluated those relationships, had come to some understanding of the reasons why her parents behaved as they did, and had made much progress in forgiving them. Finally, she described her current close and supportive relationship with her mother and her less trusting but improving relationship with her father. This mother was classified as having autonomous working models of her relationships with her parents.

Mother 2. This mother described her relationship with her own mother as stern and loving. The examples she gave for both these adjectives, however, centered on her mother's stern way of managing all the children of that generation. During this part of the interview the mother became quite anxious and confused and cried as she extensively praised her own mother in an idealizing fashion.

She described her father as easy going, always smiling, and hard working. She then went on to describe, in detail, some of the loving gestures she remembered of him from her early childhood. He seemed to have been much less rejecting of her than her mother and was the closer attachment figure. Suddenly she began to sob and told the interviewer that her father had died 9 years ago, although it seemed like yesterday. In response to questions, she described details of his sudden death, the terrible impact it had on her mother and herself, and the fact that she and her mother try not to think or talk about it because it upsets them so much. Continuing to cry, she described how her son has come to fill the void left in her mother by her father's death. Finally, she acknowledged that his death, and her refusal to think about it, must have some impact on other parts of her life. Her way of coping with it, however, is not to think about it.

This mother was classified as unresolved. It seems likely that her early insecure relationship with her mother, her not resolving and moving beyond the grief of her father's death, and her current dependence on her mother for support may all have conspired to keep her from reevaluating her early working models of close relationships. It is possible that, in turn, this has contributed significantly to her inability to resolve her son's diagnosis and keeps her from responding sensitively to his signals and needs. The final result, at this point, is that her son is neither securely attached to her nor self-reliant in exploring his world. Mother 1, on the other hand, seems to have been able to resolve her difficult early history. With this as a model, she seems to have been able to resolve her son's diagnosis, responds sensitively to him, and has successfully facilitated his development on a path toward self-reliance.

• • •

These case studies illustrate the value of studying self-reliance from a relationship and attachment perspective. They suggest the possibility of describing not only an individual child's developmental pathway toward a quality of life outcome such as self-reliance[28] but also the path that an extended family takes across a number of generations in organizing and regulating close relationships and ensuring its quality of life. Finally, this framework suggests for families of children with disabilities what Main and her colleagues have found for normal families: Specifically, unresolved, traumatic loss can have a powerful negative effect on many aspects of family functioning, especially those aspects dealing with or affected by intimate relationships. Our research goes one step further in the case of medically compromised children in that early, unresolved traumatic loss may also play a powerful negative role in parents' reactions to their children's diagnosis or in their ability to grieve successfully the loss of the perfect child. The challenge to the field of early intervention is to understand these relationship-based factors so that we will be able to develop interventions that can efficiently and effectively guide children and their families toward more functional developmental pathways.[6]

REFERENCES

1. Sabbeth B, Leventhal J. Marital adjustment to chronic childhood illness. *Pediatrics.* 1984;73:762–768.
2. Kazak A, Marvin RS. Differences, difficulties and adaptation: Stress and social networks in families with a handicapped child. *Fam Relat.* 1984;33:67–77.
3. Ainsworth MDS, Blehar MC, Waters E, Wall S. *Patterns of Attachment: A Psychological Study of the Strange Situation.* Hillsdale, NJ: Erlbaum; 1978.
4. Bowlby J. *Attachment and Loss: Attachment.* New York: Basic Books; 1969.
5. Bowlby J. *Attachment and Loss: Sadness and Depression.* New York: Basic Books; 1980;3.
6. Marvin RS, Stewart RB. A family systems framework for the study of attachment. In: Greenberg MT, Cicchetti D, Cummings EM, eds. *Attachment in the Preschool Years: Theory, Research and Intervention.* Chicago: University of Chicago Press; 1990.
7. Cicchetti D, ed. Developmental psychopathology. *Child Dev.* 1984;55.
8. Sroufe LA. Pathways to adaptation and maladaptation: Psychopathology as developmental deviation. In: Cicchetti D, ed. *The Rochester Symposium on Developmental Psychopathology.* Hillsdale, NJ: Erlbaum; 1990.
9. Greenspan S, Porges S. Psychopathology in infancy and early childhood: Clinical perspectives on the organization of sensory and affective-thematic experience. *Child Dev.* 1984;55:49–70.
10. Sameroff A, Emde R. *Relationship Disturbances in Early Childhood.* New York: Basic Books; 1988.
11. Pianta RC, Marvin RS. Procedures for assessing and classifying attachment behavior of children with moderate to severe motor impairments. Presented at the biennial meeting of the Society for Research in Child Development; April 1989; Kansas City, MO.
12. Ainsworth MDS. *Infancy in Uganda: Infant Care and the Growth of Love.* Baltimore: Johns Hopkins University Press; 1967.
13. Bowlby J. *Attachment and Loss: Separation.* New York: Basic Books; 1973;2.
14. Bretherton I. Attachment theory: Retrospect and prospect. *Monogr Soc Res Child Dev.* 1985;50:3–35.
15. Main M, Kaplan N, Cassidy J. Security in infancy, childhood and adulthood: A move to the level of representation. *Monogr Soc Res Child Dev.* 1985;50: 66–104.
16. Main M, Soloman J. Discovery of a new, insecure-disorganized/disoriented attachment pattern. In: Yogman M, Brazelton TB, eds. *Affective Development in Infancy.* Norwood, NJ: Ablex; 1986.
17. Main M, Soloman J. Procedures for identifying infants as disorganized/disoriented during the Ainsworth strange situation. In: Greenberg MT, Cicchetti D, Cummings EM, eds. *Attachment in the Preschool Years: Theory, Research and Intervention.* Chicago: University of Chicago Press; 1990.

18. Cassidy J, Marvin RS. *Attachment Organization in Two-and-One-Half to Four-and-One-Half Year-Olds: Coding Guidelines, 1992.* Charlottesville, VA: Department of Pediatrics, University of Virginia; 1992.

19. Erickson MF, Sroufe LA, Egeland B. The relationship between quality of attachment and behavior problems in preschool in a high-risk sample. *Monogr Soc Res Child Dev.* 1985 ;50:147–166.

20. Lieberman AF, Pawl JH. Disorders of attachment and secure base behavior in the second year of life: Conceptual issues and clinical intervention. In: Greenberg MT, Cicchetti D, Cummings EM, eds. *Attachment in the Preschool Years: Theory, Research and Intervention.* Chicago: University of Chicago Press; 1990.

21. Greenberg MT, DeKlyen M, Speltz M. The relationship of insecure attachment to externalizing behavior problems in the preschool years. Presented at the biennial meeting of the Society for Research in Child Development; April 1989; Kansas City, MO.

22. Goldberg S. Attachment in infants at risk: Theory, research and practice. *Infants Young Child.* 1990;2:11–20.

23. George C, Kaplan N, Main M. *The Berkeley Adult Attachment Interview.* Berkeley, CA: Department of Psychology, University of California; 1985.

24. Main M, Goldwyn R. Interview-based adult attachment classifications: Related to infant-mother and infant-father attachment. *Dev Psychol.* In press.

25. Grossman K, Frommer Bombik F, Rudolph J, Grossman KE. Maternal attachment representations as related to patterns of child-mother attachment and maternal sensitivity and acceptance of her infant. In: Hinde RA, Stevenson-Hinde J, eds. *Relations Within Families.* Oxford: Oxford University Press; 1988.

26. Fonagy P, Steele H, Steele M. Maternal representations of attachment during pregnancy predict the organization of infant-mother attachment at one year of age. *Child Dev.* 1991;62:891–905.

27. Aber L, Slade A, Berger B, Bresgi I, Kaplan M. *The Parent Development Interview.* New York: Barnard College, Columbia University; 1985.

28. Lothman D, Pianta RC, Clarson S. Mother-child interaction in children with epilepsy: Relations with child competence. *J Epilepsy.* 1990;3:157–163.

Therapy for sexually abused young children

Nitza Perlman, PhD
Psychologist

Claire Millar, MEd
Kristine Ericson, MA
Psychotherapists
Children and Youth Services
Department of Family Therapy
Surrey Place Center
Toronto, Ontario, Canada

IN RECENT YEARS there has been a proliferation of literature about the diagnosis and treatment of sexually abused children. Much of the written material in this area is retrospective; that is, it comprises accounts of adult survivors reporting their experiences of abuse as children.[1-3] There is little rigorous, scientifically based evidence for much of the published material in this area in relation to etiology, diagnosis, psychologic sequelae of the abuse, and the effectiveness and risks of the various therapies employed. The studies that do exist include methodologic problems such as various definitions of abuse and differences in the circumstances of the abuse. In addition to the above, the literature on sexual abuse seldom addresses the special needs of the young child. The little existing research on child sexual abuse predominantly addresses issues related to identification and investigation of the abuse.[4-7] In most cases, the approach adopted to treatment is influenced by clinical experience, theoretical background, and beliefs of the therapists and other caregivers. Little or no research exists attempting to analyze directly sexually abused children's understanding and perceptions of themselves, their abusers, and their experiences of the abuse. All of this calls for additional caution when decisions about interventions are made.

This article discusses the issues involved in diagnosis and treatment of young children, from preschool to latency age, who have been sexually abused. This article does not report the results of a study but rather represents the authors' recent experience with therapy of sexually abused young children. An effort has been made to incorporate a developmental perspective and to highlight problems relevant to decisions about interventions. As in other areas, when faced with an acute emergency the clinician is forced to act, making use of nonvalidated therapeutic practices based on clinical judgment.

SEXUAL ABUSE OF CHILDREN

The majority of abused young children are the victims of an older person known to them, often in the context of dependency and trust. Most of the perpetrators are fathers, foster fathers, brothers, other care providers, family members, and friends, all mostly men. The fact that the perpetrators are known to the victims raises the question of consent.

Inf Young Children 1993; 5(3): 43–48
© 1993 Aspen Publishers, Inc.

Hindman[8] states that the developmental differences between children and adults determine children's inability to consent. The inequality in the relationship makes the child's consent to an adult not possible. Children can be seduced or coerced, and the child may display seductive behavior, but the young child cannot consent because children do not have the option of refusing to participate in the particular activity. Saying no is not an option in the majority of cases. This is important not only from the legal perspective but also in terms of understanding the child's experience. The therapist and other caregivers must be aware of this issue. As work toward recovery from the trauma of the abuse progresses, the child victim will require help in accepting that he or she did not have an option, that the adult involved in the abuse was in control of the situation.

Young children with their egocentricity experience themselves both as powerless and as omnipotent. In the normal course of development, as the child grows older (and if, while he or she is growing up, all goes well), the child will learn to accept these limits. When one is supporting young children who have been abused, it is crucially important to remember that children tend to attribute the cause of events to themselves. To the child's mind, it is because of who they are and what they do that events turn out as they do. Perpetrators often exploit this developmental weakness.

In addition, young children are able to, and sometimes do, get sexually aroused. Traumatic as the experience may be in cases of abuse, aspects of the sexual contact may be gratifying for the victim. Sex offenders often talk to their victims about the victims' responsiveness, real or invented, during the sexual encounter. This behavior of the adult adds to the child's confusion and self-blame.

When, as a result of a child's disclosure, the child or another member of the family, namely the perpetrator, is removed from the home, the problems become overwhelming. In many of the reported cases, at least in the initial stages, the child is not believed; another member of the family often blames the child for the family's misfortune.

Research findings about the long-term effects of abuse are few and inconsistent. It seems clear, however, that not all abused children suffer irreversible consequences. It is therefore extremely important that a reaction to disclosure be supportive but calm. A panic response by the adult will translate in the child's mind to catastrophe. The assessment of each case has to relate to the actual events, the child's vulnerabilities, and the weaknesses and strengths of the family.

THE CHILD'S PERCEPTION OF THE ABUSE

Children perceive themselves as being in need of protection. Invariably as therapy progresses, the child has to deal with the issue of betrayal by the perpetrator and by those who knew or should have known whatever the reality was. In our clinic, the theme of the mother who failed to protect her child was introduced in therapy by almost all the abused children early in therapy. Different children express it in various ways. For example, 5-year-old Lesley locked her female therapist in an imaginary jail; the therapist was bad because she could not protect the children. Seven-year-old Paul heated food on the stove, then in the oven, and then fed it to his therapist. He wanted to burn her inside, to burn all the babies inside her; these were bad babies, and the therapist did not take care of them. The failure of the primary caregiver, the mother, to protect the child from the abuse and violation is perhaps the most damaging element in the abuse. It translates in the child's mind into a sense of not deserving to be protected, of not being worth keeping, of being worthless.

It is generally accepted that the best predictor of good outcome in the face of abuse is a solid and supportive network. A family that will stand behind the child sends a clear message that the abuse was wrong, that it was not the child's fault, and that these loving adults will do all they can to help the traumatized child. Unfortunately, it is often the case that families in which intrafamilial abuse occurs are not able to effectively support a traumatized child. Many such families have difficulties in boundary setting and observance of the boundary. These are the areas in which the sexually abused child needs help. It is therefore important that a thorough family assessment be conducted soon after the child has been referred for treatment. The purpose of the assessment is to identify major family problems that both keep family members from recognizing the perpetrator's responsibility and the perpetrator from assuming responsibility for the abuse. It also helps prevent scapegoating of the child. It is equally important to identify those areas of strength in the family that can be mobilized to support the traumatized child. Family therapy as well as individual work with the child are usually required.

It is generally accepted that when the child's safety is not in jeopardy all effort must be made so that the child can stay at home. The perpetrator, if a member of the household, should be removed or isolated from the victim. In reality, however, children are often removed from the family home as soon as disclosure occurs, in the majority of cases with no charge laid because there is little or no corroborating evidence.

After removal from the home, the child experiences extreme loss and abandonment and an acute sense of self-blame for having disclosed and thus caused the upheaval in his or her life as well as the life of the family. For the child, this becomes the ultimate confirmation of his or her badness.

FIRST STAGE OF TREATMENT: DIAGNOSIS

The most common technique used for treatment of young children is play therapy. At the initial stage, the play is used as a means of understanding the emotional condition of the child. The therapist's role in this stage is diagnostician. The assumption is that the child's play reveals what is in the child's mind in the same way that free association reveals what is in an adult's mind. When the therapist play-interacts with the child, it is for the purpose of exploring or confirming an idea about the conflicts the child is expressing and the nature of the events that caused these conflicts. This stage of assessment usually lasts more than one session because the child has to feel safe in the therapeutic setting and develop trust in the therapist. At this stage, it is important that the therapist be encouraging but not leading. By the time sexually abused children come to the attention of a trained therapist, most of them have been through extensive questioning by concerned family members, other caregivers, and the authorities. The young child is hurt, anxious, and confused. The child has disappointed an adult on whom he or she learned to be dependent. In many cases, the child is disbelieved and disvalidated, and pressure is put on the child to respond in some specific way that suits the questioning adult.

For example, Jane's mother was trying to protect the father/perpetrator by denying the disclosure. At a day-care center, a worker observed that the 4-year-old girl had vaginal bleeding. When asked about it, Jane described sexual abuse and named the father and a stepbrother as the perpetrators. The mother's response was to deny the abuse and to try to persuade Jane and the authorities that Jane had sat on broken glass. Jane was removed from the home and placed in foster care. Terrified by the changes that occurred so abruptly, she repeated the broken glass story, but crying she added "and Daddy will not do it again." Jane wanted to go home.

In the play-diagnosis interview as observed by Sgroi,[7] the therapist allows children to identify significant events in their lives and to explore their feelings about these events. This provides insight into how the abuse may affect the child's development. One tool often used in assessment of sexually abused young children is anatomically correct dolls. These are soft dolls, usually with mouth and anal openings; the females have breasts and a vaginal opening, and the males have external male genitalia. All the dolls have fingers. These dolls are supposed to provide the child with the ability to demonstrate the abusive experiences. Several writers have suggested that no conclusion about events should be drawn solely on the basis of the child's behavior with the dolls.[9,10] The child might have watched adults making love, been exposed to explicit videos, or been told about sexual activities. For instance, a mother involved in a custody battle with her husband had told her daughter with Down syndrome that she could not see her father. The father was bad because he had touched the daughter's breasts. In the session, the girl demonstrated the mother's story. No other details were given. It could of course be true, but the story was unconvincing because it lacked contextual details. On the other hand, another child mentioned the "white yakky stuff" which probably related to experience in real life.

Ideally, the therapist should not be used as an investigator for the police or the child protection authorities. This role may interfere with the therapist's relationship with other members of the family, who otherwise may be able to cooperate. It may also seriously damage the child's trusting relationship with the therapist. The therapist talking to the authorities may be seen by the child as a betrayal. The child almost always wants to be loved by, and wants to protect, the abusive family. In addition, most sexually abused children have been warned by the abuser not to tell, that something terrible will happen to them if they tell. Often the consequences of disclosure and the upheavals experienced by the family and the child are seen as confirmation of the threats. It may not be possible for a child to trust a therapist who reveals the child's secrets to the police.

In some states and in Canada the therapist may be required by law to provide the authorities with information concerning the abuse. There are also situations in which the child's safety may be in jeopardy and the therapist feels obliged to report confidential information obtained in therapy. To prevent inadvertent discovery of the therapist reporting such information, it is advisable to discuss such breaches of confidentiality with the child. An inadvertent discovery might undermine the child's trust in the therapist. The explanation to the child should focus on the therapist's concern for the child's safety rather than on punishment of the perpetrator. Although some children entertain revenge fantasies against the abuser, for the majority of young children the punishment of the perpetrator provokes a serious internal conflict.

SECOND STAGE OF TREATMENT: PLAY THERAPY

The second stage of treatment is play therapy. The therapist's focus is now not so much on the traumatizing events and the child's developmental and environmental vulnerabilities but on the fantasy material that the child presents and the symbolic meaning that these carry. It also reveals the defenses employed by the young child in the face of the traumatic events.

Freud[11] was the first to describe play as an attempt to master a traumatizing situation. Freud observed an 18-month-old boy repeatedly throwing a toy away from himself and then pulling it back. Freud interpreted this game as an exercise in mastery of the anxiety associated with the mother's disappearances from the world that the child perceives. In play, the child becomes an active participant. He or she experiments through play, mastering the situation. Therapy actually works when the therapist has created, in the session room, a situation safe enough that the child can afford to "let the demons out" and, through the play, to reenact the confusing and anxiety-producing events. It is then that the therapist must be able to enter the child's play.[12] Direct interpretations relating the content of the play to real-life situations will strip the ego of its defenses. It can be experienced as a direct attack on the immature and fragile ego of the young child. The therapist joins the child's play, the child's fantasy. Only later, when the themes have been reenacted several times, will the therapist carefully choose the time for interpreting.

Four-year-old Linda brought a baby doll from home to the treatment center. She would enter the room and drop the doll on the floor. No one was allowed to pick the "baby" up. For several sessions, the therapist reflected, "No one is taking care of this baby. It must feel very bad not to be looked after properly." After these sessions, the therapist suggested, "It must have been difficult for you when your parents did not know how to properly take care of you." After that, Linda placed the baby doll in a crib. The baby doll was never mistreated again.

In play therapy, the therapist must be trusted and the child must feel safe in the session room so as to promote the condition in which it is relatively safe to reenact the traumatizing events. By repeating the frightening theme, the child can be desensitized, to some extent, to the anxiety associated with the theme played. More importantly, in play, the child has some opportunity to be active, not just a victim.

The process of working through these issues in therapy is illustrated in the following cases. Five-year-old Sheila, upon entering the play therapy room, would arrange the chairs in a row. The therapist was the driver of this "chair-train." The same doll, called by the patient Little Sheila, was put in a little cot on one of the chairs and covered carefully. This was so that the guards would not find her, she explained. The therapist's purse was also used as a hiding place for babies. Sheila repeated that theme for six sessions. Jane, for the first three sessions, was riding a tricycle and ordered the therapist to push the big car and follow her. "Hurry! Hurry!" she said to the therapist. "We must find all the little boys and girls, they are afraid, they are hiding, find them, hurry!" Three-year-old Craig would start many sessions by selecting all the toys ("babies") and throwing them furiously out of the room with "You are bad; get out." Elizabeth, early in therapy, described herself as sitting on the roof, alone; she was afraid, and there was no one there with her. Two sessions later she said that the therapist was with her on the roof. At the next session, the same theme was repeated; she was on the roof again, but not alone anymore. The therapist and her foster mother were with her, and she was not so afraid anymore.

•   •   •

Play therapy enables abused children to convey their experiences—their internal reality—and, with the help of the therapist, to work through some of the traumatizing aspects of the abuse. The therapist provides a safe and trustworthy environment. By interpreting the play themes, the therapist helps the child organize his or her experiences and validates for the child his or her emotional response. The child is not so alone anymore in his or her fear and despair. Nevertheless, the problem of child sexual abuse is not going to go away. What is badly needed is disciplined outcome research that will guide the clinician in deciding about interventions.

REFERENCES

1. Courtois C. *Healing the Incest Wound: Adult Survivor in Therapy.* 1st ed. New York: Norton; 1988.
2. Goodwin J. *Sexual Abuse: Incest Victims and their Families.* Chicago: Year Book Medical; 1989.
3. Herman JL. *Father-Daughter Incest.* Cambridge, Mass: Harvard University Press; 1981.
4. Gale J, Thompson RJ, Moran T, Sack WH, William H. Sexual abuse in young children: Its clinical presentation and characteristic patterns. *Child Abuse Neg.* 1988;12:163–170.
5. Goldston DB, Turnguist DC, Knutson JF. Presenting problems of sexually abused girls receiving psychiatric services. *J Abnorm Psychol.* 1989;3:314–317.
6. Miller T, Veltkamp LJ, Jason D. Projective measures in the clinical evaluation of sexually abused children. *Child Psychiat Hum Dev.* 1987; 18:47–57.
7. Sgroi SM. *Vulnerable Populations: Evaluation and Treatment of Sexually Abused Children and Adult Survivors.* Lexington, Mass: Lexington Books; 1985.
8. Hindman J. *Just Before Dawn: From the Shadows of Tradition to New Reflections in Trauma Assessment and Treatment of Sexual Victimization.* Boise, Idaho: Northwest Printing; 1989.
9. Everson MD, Boat BW. Sexualized doll play among young children: Implications for the use of anatomical dolls in sexual abuse evaluations. *J Am Acad Child Adolesc Psychiatr.* 1990;29:736–742.
10. Yates A, Terr L. Anatomically correct dolls: Should they be used as the basis for expert testimony? *J Am Acad Child Adolesc Psychiatr.* 1988;27:254–257.
11. Freud S. Beyond the pleasure principle. In: *The Standard Edition of the Complete Psychological Works of Sigmund Freud.* London: Hogarth; 1955:18.
12. Winnicott DW. *Playing and Reality.* Harmondsvorth, Penguin; 1971.

Early intervention for infants and toddlers with prenatal drug exposure

Fay F. Russell, MN, RN(C)
Coordinator of Early Intervention and
   Chief of Nursing
Boling Center for Developmental
   Disabilities
Associate Professor
Health Sciences Center
University of Tennessee–Memphis
Memphis, Tennessee

Teresa A. Free, PhD, RN(C)
Assistant Professor
University of Kentucky College of
   Nursing
Lexington, Kentucky

AT LEAST ONE of every ten newborns in the United States (approximately 400,000 infants) is exposed to illegal substances during the gestational period.[1] In addition, two to six children per 1000 suffer effects from exposure to legal alcohol.[2] A recent study[3] in Florida suggested that there is little difference in the prevalence of drug and alcohol use between prenatal patients at private and public health care facilities. Children exposed to these potentially harmful substances during the vulnerable developmental period before birth often grow up in a childhood environment where the mother continues to abuse drugs and where there are limited mother–child interactions and learning experiences, placing the infant at both biological and environmental risk.[4]

The child exposed to drugs in utero presents a constellation of physical, developmental, and behavioral effects the severity of which depends on the chemical substance and dosage. Children whose mothers drank alcohol during pregnancy may exhibit facial defects that include eye aberrations (eg, short palpebral fissures, strabismus, ptosis), broad flattened nasal bridges with short upturned noses, flattened philtrums, hypoplastic upper lips, and micrognathia.[5] Inadequate growth of the head and body are clinically recognized as microcephaly and microsomia. Infants demonstrate irritability, hypotonia, and a dose-related range of developmental delays. Mothers who drink heavily risk having a child with fetal alcohol syndrome, which is manifested by many or all of the above physical defects and by mild to moderate mental retardation.

Marijuana and cocaine are the most common illicit substances used by childbearing women. Marijuana has been associated with neonatal tremors, exaggerated startle responses, and altered visual functioning, but no characteristic physical features.[6] Cocaine and "crack," an inexpensive and very addictive form of cocaine, are highly associated with severe perinatal insults and central nervous

This project was supported by OHDS Grant No. 04-DD-000167 from the Administration on Developmental Disabilities. Additional support was provided by MCH Training Grant No. 000900, Maternal and Child Health Bureau, US Dept of Health and Human Services.
The authors acknowledge the assistance of Gerald Golden, MD, Donna Hathaway, PhD, Mary Todd, MSSW, and Judith Powell, MPH.

system dysfunction. Cocaine causes vasoconstriction, tachycardia, and acute hypertension in the mother and restricted blood flow, tachycardia, and hyperactivity in the fetus. These insults can lead to first trimester abortion, abruptio placentae, premature labor, fetal cerebral infarctions, and stillbirths. The physiological and behavioral consequences for the infant who survives these insults may be extreme irritability, jitteriness, tremors, seizures, hypertonia, tachycardia, tachypnea, abnormal respiratory patterns, difficulty feeding, and abnormal sleep patterns.[1,7] As the infant becomes a toddler, he or she may experience speech and language deficits, play differences, and flat emotional reactions.[8]

Identifying the deficits produced by specific drugs has been problematic. Most chronic substance-abusing women identify a drug of choice but actually engage in polydrug use. Since the effects of multiple drugs are cumulative, polydrug use makes it difficult to identify what outcomes are related to specific drugs.

UNDERSTANDING ALCOHOL AND DRUG ADDICTION

It is sometimes difficult for health care professionals to understand why women use harmful substances during their pregnancy and place their unborn child at risk for permanent damage. Denial, a major element of addiction, and family dynamics appear to be important contributing factors to this destructive process. The woman who uses chemical substances during pregnancy cannot actually see the effects of drugs on the developing fetus, and her craving for the drug overtakes any fear of danger to herself or her child. Even after the child is born with physical and behavioral problems, the mother's resumption of alcohol or drug use enables her to escape the consequences of her actions. The escape may be intentional on the mother's part or a secondary effect of the drug-induced blunting of emotions.

Family dynamics, or "family trap" described by Wegsheider-Cruse,[9] constitute the roles family members assume to cope with addiction. The chemically dependent parent is the central focus of the family. The spouse usually becomes the chief enabler by helping the abuser function in daily life despite the addiction. As chief enabler, the spouse may even assist the abuser's acquisition of drugs by providing financial support and making excuses for missed workdays. These behaviors of the enabling spouse are referred to as "codependence," a preoccupation or extreme emotional and social dependency with the abuser. The children's roles also are affected by the family disease. One child, most often the oldest, becomes the "hero," an overachiever and nurturer, who may emulate the chief enabler. Another child becomes the scapegoat, whose behaviors cause problems at home and school and resemble the substance-using parent. Two other roles children may assume are the lost child or the mascot. The lost child, who is isolated and uninformed about family matters, is at special risk for addiction. The mascot, the lovable clown, entertains the family to get attention. Children's roles may vacillate, and a combination of the above roles may be seen in each individual. An only child may intermittently demonstrate all four roles. Each role balances the others; therefore, a change in any one family member's role could have a tremendous impact on the entire family.[9]

An environment of poverty often accompanies the dynamics of this dysfunctional family. The impoverished environment compounds family dysfunction by creating situations that demand additional problem solving and coping by family members. When coping behaviors are inadequate, dysfunction is accentuated.

In single parent families, the codependency relationship may develop between the addicted mother and her own mother. The grandmother experiences shame, guilt, and immense responsibility for the disappointing behavior of her daughter and feels compelled to see that her grandchildren do not suffer. To accomplish this, the grandmother frequently assumes care of the children. Sometimes the mother lives with the grandmother and relates to her own children as if she were their sibling, relying on the grandmother for daily feeding, clothing, and safety of the children. Other mothers may literally be "on the streets" or incarcerated; the grandmother rescues the children from foster care by taking them into her home. Both patterns diminish the mother's child-care responsibilities, enabling her to continue drug and alcohol use, whether it be weekend binge-drinking or chronic everyday use. If the grandmother or other adult family members are unable or unwilling to care for the children, an older child often assumes responsibility for younger siblings.

Within this family trap, the children of addicted parents are hidden victims. They experience low self-esteem and emotional trauma. The double messages they receive from their addicted parent preclude the development of a trust relationship. As the children of addicts grow older, they may also experience physical neglect as they are left in the care of other children or even left to care for themselves. Health care is not a priority and often is neglected. Safety and accident prevention in the home rarely receive attention. The risks of physical abuse and emotional neglect are increased for children in the addicted family.[9,10]

Families in the trap of addiction, whether intact or not, are often severely dysfunctional and resistant to change. Family members learn to manipulate the care system, always having excuses for their noncompliance with health maintenance or treatment recommendations. Minimizing, rationalizing, and lying are coping strategies the family uses to meet demands or expectations of the outside world.

Addiction has been described as a multigenerational problem with genetic and environmental variables thought to be causative factors. In most families of a substance-using mother, extended family members are also heavy drinkers or drug users. This environment of addiction undoubtedly contributes to high failure rates for rehabilitation of substance users.[9]

EARLY INTERVENTION FOR FAMILIES WITH ADDICTION

Philosophical framework

In 1987 an interdisciplinary team at the University of Tennessee–Memphis, Boling Center for Developmental Disabilities undertook the development of a new early intervention program (EIP) to serve infants and toddlers with prenatal drug exposure and their families. The program was initiated in response to the growing number of children born to substance-using women in Memphis. The child-care support and addiction-recovery services required by the families of these substance-exposed children were overwhelming existing health and social service delivery systems. Two major national trends guided the philosophical direction and approach: Public Law 99-457, the Education for the Handicapped Law Amendments of 1986, authorizing early intervention services for handicapped infants and toddlers and their families, and the national upsurge in alcohol and drug use, particularly cocaine, in pregnant women. The team believed that an effective early intervention program for the children and their caregivers should incorporate four criteria: (1) an interdisciplinary approach from the field of developmental disabilities for services with families of young children, (2) case management based on Individualized Family Service Plans (IFSPs), (3) health and social services that address the needs of substance-exposed children and dysfunctional families, and (4) clarification of values and cultural sensitivity of team members.

Program assumptions

This early intervention program was based on the following assumptions:
- Children identified as having prenatal drug exposure are at high risk for physical, intellectual, emotional, or social delays capable of interfering with normal growth, development, and learning capacity.
- An enriching home environment improves the child's development and social adjustment.
- Parenting skills of parents or caregivers are enhanced through knowledge in all areas of normal development and childrearing.

Program goals

The goals of this early intervention program were fourfold:
1. Enrolled children would benefit by their families' enhanced ability to provide an environment that nurtured physical, social, emotional, and cognitive development.

2. The substance abuser's motivation to seek treatment and rehabilitation would be strengthened, decreasing the probability that subsequent children will be exposed prenatally to drugs.
3. Families would gain a better understanding of addiction and its effects on individuals and families.
4. Team members working with this population would acquire a specialized body of knowledge and skills and would disseminate this information to students and other professionals.

Strategies for intervention

The early planning team consisted of professionals interested in drug-exposed children and included representatives from nursing, pediatrics, genetics, social work, speech pathology and audiology, nutrition, physical therapy, and psychology. The program was initiated by a team comprising nurses, social workers, a nutritionist, a physical therapist, a speech pathologist, and an audiologist. A clinical nursing specialist experienced in early intervention directed the project.

High priority was given to training the team in treating the disease of alcohol and drug addiction. Training required three 4-hour sessions and was provided by a specialist in alcohol and drug counseling. Content included the addiction disease process, the roles family members assume, codependency, and support for families in recovery. Although team members did not intend to provide direct rehabilitation services, they needed to know when to direct families to recovery programs and how to support the recovery process.

Armed with experiences from a previously successful early intervention program[11] and the alcohol and drug training, the EIP team began the planning phase. Activities were planned for a family program composed of ten 4-hour weekly sessions. Time for family assessment, developmental assessment, interventions, evaluations, and follow-up were included. Incentives for participation were built into the program and included transportation for the families to the center (a major expense), a nutritious snack and lunch for parents or caregivers and children, and a gift such as a developmental toy or safety product. Before beginning the center-based program, each family received a home visit by an EIP team nurse. This visit was used for developmental screening and to complete the Home Observation of the Environment (HOME) scale, The Nursing Child Assessment Teaching Scales (NCATS), and The Nursing Child Assessment Feeding Scales (NCAFS).[12] The HOME scale was used to measure the stimulation potential of the child's immediate environment. Both the NCATS and NCAFS test the ability of the infant to produce clear cues and to respond to his or her caregiver. The abilities of the parent or caregiver to respond to the infant's cues, to alleviate distress, and to create growth-fostering situations was assessed using the nursing child assessment scales. The home visit also helped prepare the families for the early intervention experiences.

Social workers from the Regional Medical Center Newborn Division and nurses from the Memphis and Shelby County Health Department identified and referred appropriate families who were willing to participate. The majority of participants were inner-city, low-income (54, 93%), black (57, 98%) families. The mothers were typically in their late 20s, and the grandmothers' ages ranged from 40 to 65 years. Sixty-one (86%) of the children were born to mothers who were single. Each family was expected to attend 10 weekly sessions. The child and primary caregivers were invited. After the home visit, 44 (76%) of the families participated in at least two sessions, 34 (58%) participated in at least 5 sessions, and 21 (36%) participated in 8 or more sessions. Over 2½ years, seven ten-week programs were conducted and 59 families served. It was common for parents and caregivers to be excited and enthusiastic during the referral and home visit process and then find excuses not to attend, a typical behavior of addictive families.

Table 1 outlines a typical 10-week program, including the topics for parent or caregiver training, the incentives to be distributed, and the support group themes. Specific activities for a typical four-hour session are seen in Fig 1. Ten to 15 families were enrolled for each program. Telephone calls were made weekly before each program session to encourage attendance and clarify transportation plans.

Parents or caregivers spent approximately 2½ hours each week in training and support groups. At least four sessions were spent sharing information about addiction, codependency, and recovery. A very important part of the support groups was the consistent attendance of a volunteer who was a recovering alcoholic and mother of two older children with fetal alcohol syndrome. Her disclosure of her own illness and recovery facilitated group participation.

Early in the sessions, assessments were completed on the children that included history and physical examination, audiological assessment, speech–language screening, and nutrition and feeding assessments. For children who scored below age level on the developmental screening performed in the home, further developmental assessment was done. Following assessments, infants and toddlers were assigned planned developmental and learning activities. For infants, most activities were individually implemented. For toddlers, groups of two or three children provided the best approach for the learning or developmental activity.

Case management services and the IFSP, both specific components of Public Law 99-457, were adapted and implemented for this early intervention program. Case management was conceptualized as a collaborative endeavor of families and professionals focused on planning interventions for children with special needs. Case management involves advocating for families and interfacing with larger community systems for planning, facilitating, monitoring, follow-up, and quality assurance of services within the planned intervention (Burgess E. May 1990. Per-

Table 1. Ten-week schedule of activities for early intervention program

Session number	Parent or caregiver group training	Attendance incentive	Support group topic
1	Introductions Overview of program	Gift pack of product samples, booklets, and personal items	Forms completed and signed
2	Preventive health care for children	Thermometer	Child development knowledge pretest
3	Safety in the home	Electrical outlet cover Coloring book	Chemical dependency: The disease concept
4	Child-growth and motor development	Blocks or rattle	The family disease
5	Learning through play	Book made by parent or caregiver	Codependency
6	Child speech– Language and Communication	Mirror or toy telephone	Recovery
7	Nutrition and feeding	Bib and spoon Placemat	Self esteem
8	Self-care skills	Teething ring Dental kit	Assertiveness
9	Psychosocial development	Photograph of child in frame	Stress management
10	Behavior management	Child's chair	Goal setting Child development knowledge posttest Evaluation of experience

sonal communication). One EIP team member was assigned to each family as case manager with responsibility for supporting the family through the EIP process, introducing the family to other members of the team, documenting the family and child's progress, and identifying and supporting the family's use of appropriate community resources. The case manager and family collaborated to develop the IFSP, which helps the family identify their strengths and needs and those of their child, sets appropriate goals, priorities and time frames, and identifies the best available resources to meet the goals.[13] The IFSP process culminates in a written document of child and family assessments, established goals, and strategies for goal achievement. In this EIP, weekly conferences with the family and case manager included discussion of progress toward the goals.

Session No _____

Time	Activity	Participants
8:30–8:45	Preconference	Interdisciplinary team
8:45–9:00	Families arrive	Case managers
	Nametags for everyone	Families
	Label all belongings	
	Coffee for parents or caregivers	
9:00–10:15	Parent or caregiver group training	Parents or caregivers
		Assigned team member
	Planned developmental activities	Infants and toddlers
	Individual and group	Team members
		Trainees and volunteers
	Complete speech–language screening	Speech pathologist
10:15–10:30	Break	Parents or caregivers
	Potty, snacks	Children
		Parents or caregivers
		Infants and toddlers
		Team members
10:340–12:00	Support group	Parents or caregivers
		Group leaders
10:40–1:00	Developmental activities and lunch	Children
		Assigned team members
12:00–12:30	Lunch	Parents or caregivers
		Group leaders
12:30–1:00	Case management	Case managers meet with families
1:00	Families depart	
1:00–2:00	Post-Conference	Interdisciplinary team

Fig 1. Sample early intervention schedule.

Families with addiction in EI programs

Families of addiction were found to differ substantially from families with Down syndrome infants that had been served by the authors' previous EIP. Nearly 100% of the infants with Down syndrome were in the care of their natural mothers, but only 44 (62%) of the substance-exposed children were in the care of their biological mothers. The remaining children were in the care of grandmothers (17), maternal aunts (4), great grandmother (1), great aunt (1), adoptive parents (1), foster parents (2), and a nonrelative (1). Of the 44 children being cared for by their mothers, 19 actually were living with their mother in their grandmother's home, and the grandmother participated significantly in the child's care.

Unlike the parents of children with the Down syndrome, parents and caregivers from the families with addiction did not anticipate developmental lags or deviations in their children. Denial or distraction to other problems may have contributed to this phenomenon. Instead, parents and caregivers sought respite from the care of their children and were focused on their own social, health, and interpersonal needs. The parents of children with the Down syndrome valued hands-on and verbal interaction experiences in the early intervention program. In contrast, substance using mothers often sat in periods of silence when working with their children. One-word commands were common. Social interaction with another adult seemed preferable to interaction with their children. Because of these differences, the tactic of building on positive parent–child interactions, which had worked with parents of children with Down syndrome, could rarely be employed with families with addiction. Before steps could be taken to strengthen the caregiver–infant interaction and encourage the child's development, parent and caregiver needs had to be addressed. In many instances, the ten weekly sessions were nearing completion by the time parents and caregivers could attend to the needs of their children.

The traditional "deficit model" or "match model" approaches to work with families have focused on family problems or weaknesses. Using the IFSP, the case manager and family collaborate in identifying the child and family strengths as well as needs, and family goals must be based on family strengths. This was a change in focus for families as well as case managers. Families responded positively to empowerment, which was actualized by giving encouragement and assistance in pursuing goals that were outgrowths of strengths. Close emotional attachments to their children, a common strength, was used to encourage families to acquire services that the children needed. One client's strength of being motivated toward self-reliance was used to encourage the goal of acquiring independent housing.

Outcomes

To measure the first goal of the early intervention program, developmental progress and family needs are monitored annually. Attendance incentives, acquired through participation in the EIP, have given the children added learning opportunities. Participation in the EIP support groups resulted in client reports of having a new understanding of addiction and its effects on families. However, increased motivation toward recovery by substance users could not be documented. Enhanced self-esteem was reflected in improved affect and appearance. Case managers estimate that 25% of the parents and caregivers were able to identify the problems of their children more realistically. The families identified the emotional and social support of the case managers as the major strength of the early intervention program.

An important outcome for the interdisciplinary EIP team has been the acquisition of unique knowledge and skills for working with substance-exposed children and families with addiction, which have become the basis of an Early Intervention Training Project.

Follow-up

Transition plans for each family were developed by the case manager in collaboration with the family and EIP team. Children with developmental delays were referred to other early intervention programs, preschools, or Head Start.[14] Identified health problems were referred to the child's primary care clinic or to a specialty clinic. Family members were referred for assistance to community service agencies. When readiness for recovery was determined, family members were helped to identify community treatment services (ie, Alcoholics Anonymous, Narcotics Anonymous, Al-Anon). Most parents or caregivers knew of available primary care health services but used them inappropriately. For example, some children with upper respiratory infections were taken to an emergency room for treatment rather than a clinic, and many children were not adequately immunized. A frequent goal on the IFSPs was that the child receive scheduled wellness and intermittent illness care from a consistent primary health care provider.

Families who participated in the ten-week early intervention program are seen annually for a family needs assessment; at this time, children have a physical examination and developmental assessment. These annual assessments, conducted in one of the center's clinics, are scheduled during the month of the child's birth until their fifth birthday. Approximately 50% of families keep these appointments. Those who fail to attend the clinic are referred to public health nurses for follow-up care.

•   •   •

New program planners should consider building a strong and well-defined system for measuring the developmental progress of children before and after a specific period of intervention. Measures that reflect the effect of the program on substance users' seeking and achieving sobriety are needed. Research that evaluates the long-term effects of substance abuse on prenatally exposed children and the family of early intervention participants will facilitate program planning by specialists in early intervention.

REFERENCES

1. Schneider JW, Griffith DR, Chasnoff IJ. Infants exposed to cocaine in utero: Implications for developmental assessment and intervention. *Inf Young Children.* 1989;2(1):25–36.
2. Abel EL. Consumption of alcohol during pregnancy: A review of effects on growth and development of offspring. *Hum Biol.* 1982;54:421–453.
3. Chasnoff IJ, Landress HJ, Barrett ME. The prevalence of illicit-drug or alcohol use during pregnancy and discrepancies in mandatory reporting in Pinellas County, Florida. *N Engl J Med.* 1990;322:1202–1206.

4. Aylward GP. Environmental influences on the developmental outcome of children at risk. *Inf Young Children.* 1990;2(4):1–9.

5. Petrakis PL. *Alcohol and Birth Defects. The Fetal Alcohol Syndrome and Related Disorders.* Rockville, Md: US Dept of Health and Human Services; 1987. Publication ADM 87–1531.

6. Fried PA. Postnatal consequences of maternal marijuana use. *National Institute on Drug Abuse Research Monograph Series.* 1985;59:61–72.

7. Lewis KD, Bennett B, Schmeder NH. The care of infants menaced by cocaine abuse. *Am J Maternal Child Nurs.* 1989;14:324–329.

8. Howard J. Cocaine and its effects on the newborn. *Dev Med Child Neurol.* 1989;31:255–257.

9. Wegscheider-Cruse S. *Another Chance: Hope and Health for the Alcoholic Family.* 2nd ed. Palo Alto, Calif: Science and Behavior Books; 1989.

10. Einstein S. The ecology of drug use: Considerations for intervention planning. *Int J Addictions.* 1985;20:1443–1449.

11. Connolly BH, Morgan S, Russell FF. Evaluation of children with Down syndrome who participated in an early intervention program: Second follow-up study. *Phys Ther.* 1984;64:1515–1519.

12. Barnard K. *Nursing Child Assessment Teaching Scale.* Seattle, Wash: University of Washington School of Nursing, 1978.

13. Johnson BH, McGonigel MJ, Kaufmann RK, eds. *Guidelines and Recommended Practices for the Individualized Family Service Plan.* Washington, DC. Association for the Care of Children's Health; 1989.

14. Free TA, Russell FF, Mills BC, Hathaway D. A descriptive study of infants and toddlers exposed prenatally to substance abuse. *Am J Maternal Child Nurs.* 1990;15:245–249.

Consultation: Applications to early intervention

Patsy P. Coleman, MS, CCC-SLP
Speech–Language Pathologist
Carolina Literacy Center

Virginia Buysse, MS, ECSE
Research Associate
Frank Porter Graham Child
    Development Center
University of North Carolina at
    Chapel Hill
Chapel Hill, North Carolina

Dale L. Scalise-Smith, MS, LPT
Physical Therapist
Frank Porter Graham Child
    Development Center

Ann C. Schulte, PhD
Assistant Professor
Frank Porter Graham Child
    Development Center

IN THE FACE of critical personnel shortages and increasing demands for health-related personnel,[1-4] alternatives to direct child-centered delivery of early intervention services must be considered for successful implementation of Part H of IDEA (Individuals with Disabilities Act), formerly Public Law 99-457.[4,5] Consultation, an indirect approach where early interventionists work with families and other professionals to increase their independent functioning with infants and toddlers with special needs, is an appropriate option to be included in service delivery programs. The triadic nature of consultation makes effective use of available personnel, but, like all aspects of early intervention, should be used according to the needs and preferences of families.

A rich history of consultation exists in fields such as psychology, social work, and counseling, but the process has not been specifically addressed in early intervention. Although professionals working in early intervention have used consultation, this service delivery option can be greatly enhanced by borrowing from the shared experience of other fields that have broad-based descriptions of and research-oriented support for the consultative framework.

The purposes of this article are to define and describe consultation as it is used in the mental health fields and to apply this service delivery option to work with families in early intervention. Consulting with other professionals and paraprofessionals is certainly an effective use of early intervention personnel, and is the topic of several other articles.[6,7] This article concludes with a case study of a child receiving early intervention services and an example of a family-focused problem identification interview using consultative verbal processes.

The authors thank Don Bailey and Pam Winton for reviewing an earlier draft of this manuscript.

Inf Young Children 1991; 4(2): 41–46
© 1991 Aspen Publishers, Inc.

CONSULTATION DEFINED

Consultation is broadly defined in the psychological literature as an indirect problem-solving process where a consultant (early interventionist) and a consultee (caregiver) work together to define a problem and bring about its resolution.[8] Consultation is an indirect process because the consultant indirectly helps to solve a client's (child's) problems by working with a consultee who directly works with the client. This triadic nature of consultation provides skills that enable the consultee to do most of the direct work and to deal with similar problems in the future. The need for the consultant to devote time in current and future direct service delivery is reduced. Consultation is an empowering, help-giving process resulting in increased independent functioning of consultees and clients,[9] thereby reducing the need for consultants in the future.

In addition to helping to alleviate the need for some service delivery personnel, several tenets of consultation meet many of the standards described as best practice in early intervention.[10,11] The basic assumptions of consultation found throughout the psychological literature that apply to best practice in early intervention include

- proactive emphasis on the prevention of problems;
- proactive enlargement of the consultee's view to see children with special needs rather than "problem" children, strengths rather than deficits (delays/needs) can then be used in problem resolution;
- enablement of consultants and consultees to understand the larger picture of factors, such as family situations, that may be affecting a child's behavior and development; and
- empowerment of consultees to use skills provided through consultation to solve future difficulties on their own.

In response to child and family needs, the indirect, proactive, and enabling approach used in consultation can be an appropriate alternative to direct service delivery in early intervention that will effectively and efficiently use available personnel. Consultation fits well with certain aspects of Part H, PL 99-457, that require professionals from a variety of backgrounds to work together with families and other professionals to provide services to young children with special needs and their families .

THE CONSULTATIVE APPROACH AND APPLICATIONS TO EARLY INTERVENTION

There are several approaches to consultation in the mental health fields (eg, behavioral, mental health, systems), but, in general, consultation is viewed as a problem-solving process with several common steps: problem identification, problem analysis, plan implementation, and problem evaluation. As a clearly defined problem-solving model, consultation is advantageous to personnel from a wide variety of disciplines working together and working with families in early intervention.

The goal of consultation is to change the child's behavior in a desired fashion.[12] After discussing a family's need to help the child achieve specific skills and behaviors, the first step in achieving change is for the consultant and the consultee to define a problem in behavioral terms. A problem (medical, developmental, behavioral issues) is defined as the discrepancy between current and desired behaviors. This process is completed by determining environmental events and medical/developmental issues surrounding a behavior.

During consultative interviews, the consultant uses specific verbal processes to determine the nature of the problem. These processes include questions to specify the problem in behavioral terms, to indicate surrounding events, and to validate a consultant's reflection of the consultees' concerns. Consultants also use summary statements that summarize and reflect what consultees are saying in their own words. Examples of these verbal processes are included in the case study below.

The consultant and consultee then work together to devise a plan to observe and record instances of the behavior to better understand preceding, subsequent, and consequent events. From this information, the consultant helps the consultee to develop a plan of action to change the behavior to a desired outcome. The consultee (caregiver) is responsible for plan implementation. Consultation is completed when both the consultant and consultee are satisfied that behavioral objectives have been achieved.

Consultee acceptance of the implementation plan and behavioral objectives is enhanced by his or her participation and input into the behavioral consultation process. Consultees are asked to contribute information on strategies that they have tried and on the level of success or failure of a particular strategy. Consultees are also encouraged to develop plans to gather needed data. Most important, consultees assist in developing a plan of implementation that best suits their particular situation.

This emphasis on collaboration between the consultant and consultees (caregivers) in defining and solving problems reflects best practice in early intervention service delivery. When parents are not involved in setting goals for themselves, they may feel pressure to engage in an activity or work toward a goal recommended by an "expert," despite the fact that they do not believe it to be important.[13] The collaborative approach of consultation may help to ameliorate this problem.

Like family-focused practice in early intervention,[10] the consultative approach addresses the concerns outlined by the consultees (caregivers), not necessarily consultants. Limited success in traditional parent-training models has been realized, because the parent's agenda was not considered in plan development.[14] Strategy implementation by consultees, families, and other professionals is greatly increased through the collaborative problem identification and plan development process used in consultation.[8]

In addition to encouraging active consultee participation in problem definition and solution development to increase successful plan implementation, consultation also promotes self-efficacy in consultees.[8] Feelings of self-efficacy, or the confidence that one can perform the task at hand, are developed when the consultee successfully implements the plan which he or she and the consultant have developed.[8] As previously mentioned, successful plan implementation is determined when both the consultant and consultee are satisfied with the results.

The consultative approach increases the independent functioning of families and other caregivers by helping them to identify problematic areas in behavioral terms and to develop workable strategies to either increase or decrease behaviors. This collaborative problem-solving process helps build a consultee's feelings of self-efficacy. This approach to service delivery, when kept flexible to meet the needs of individual families, can enable and empower the consultees—a major goal of early intervention services.[10]

CASE STUDY

This case study was developed to illustrate how the principles of consultation outlined above may be applied to work with families in early intervention. The case itself represents a composite of several children and families and provides a brief medical history and a description of pertinent background information. A portion of a consultative interview, in which the consultant uses specific verbal processes to facilitate collaborative problem solving, appears in Table 1.

Jennifer was born during the 30th week of gestation, weighing 1,000 g, or about 2 lb, at birth. Jennifer's mother, a high school student residing with her mother and three younger siblings, was 15 years old at the time of Jennifer's birth. Jennifer spent the first 3 months of her life in the neonatal intensive care unit, where she suffered from respiratory distress syndrome, a grade III intraventricular hemorrhage, and bouts of apnea and bradycardia.

During a 3-month follow-up visit to the Special Infant Care Clinic, Jennifer's physician informed her family that Jennifer's medical history, along with her irritability, poor suck, delayed motor development, and muscle hypertonia, could be attributed to a mild form of cerebral palsy. Regular physical therapy treatments were recommended and implemented, but Jennifer's family had difficulty following through because of transportation problems.

After a 12-month follow-up visit to a regional center for developmental evaluation, Jennifer was referred by her physician to the Special Infant Care Clinic. Jennifer's mother and grandmother expressed an interest in home-based early in-

Table 1. Verbal processes used during family consultation

Dialogue	Consultant's focus
Consultant: You've asked to meet with me today to discuss some concerns you have about Jennifer. Before beginning our discussion about Jennifer, let's talk a little bit about how we should proceed. I would like to see us participating equally in developing a plan to meet Jennifer's needs as well as your needs as a family. You two know Jennifer better than anyone else. The information that you can provide is extremely important in determining what's best for Jennifer.	Role structuring/ relationship building
Let's begin by having you tell me how things are going with Jennifer.	Seeks background information
Mother: I'm not sure what Jennifer should be doing. She seems to have problems moving around and she isn't saying any words yet.	
Grandmother: My other grandchildren could walk by now. She seems like she would like to, but I don't know.	
Consultant: You seem to have several concerns about Jennifer, including her difficulty in moving and her limited speech. Is that right?	Seeks validation
Mother: Right, because she either sits there or one of us has to carry her around all day.	
Consultant: All right, it sounds like the thing you're most concerned about is that Jennifer is not getting around the way other children her age do.	Narrows the focus and validates the problem
Mother: Uh-huh.	
Consultant: When you put some toys just out of her reach, will Jennifer try to move towards them?	Specifies target behaviors
Grandmother: Jennifer really doesn't move by herself. Someone always brings the toys to her.	
Consultant: How do you feel about someone always carrying Jennifer?	Assesses the impact on family members
Mother: Well, I know it's not good for Jennifer to be so dependent on others.	
Grandmother: Yeah! And I'm afraid she's not going to learn like she's supposed to, because of these physical problems.	
Consultant: Well then, one of your goals for Jennifer might be for her to move independently around the house. Is that what you're thinking about?	Seeks validation
Mother: Yeah, but how?	
Consultant: Well, in my experience with children like Jennifer, many have learned to walk, scoot, or use special equipment to move around.	Provides information
Let's see, have you ever seen Jennifer move by herself?	Determines current skills

continues

Table 1. continued

Dialogue	Consultant's focus
Grandmother: Last week when I went to answer the phone, I cam back and found that Jennifer had moved off the blanket. I don't know how she did it. I've never actually seen her move toward anything. Do you think she could have rolled off?	
Consultant: Yes! It sounds like Jennifer is beginning to move on her own. That's good.	Affirms caregiver's observation
I think that it might be important for us to watch for other attempts to move independently. What do you think?	Seeks validation
Mother: Okay. Maybe Jennifer can move more than we think she can.	
Grandmother: Uh-huh.	
Mother: But I'm not sure what to expect from her.	
Consultant: Well how would you like to see Jennifer getting around at home?	Seeks specification of desired behavioral outcome
Mother: I want her to be able to walk!	
Consultant: Well, for now, would you like to see Jennifer moving independently and playing with her toys and work towards her walking?	Summarizes family's desired outcome
Mother: That would be wonderful!!	

tervention services. They were especially concerned about Jennifer's motor and language development. An early interventionist met with Jennifer's caregivers to determine collaborative goals as part of the process in establishing an individualized family service plan.

The consultative interview helped Jennifer's mother, grandmother and the consultant (early interventionist) to more clearly identify their goals and priorities for Jennifer. After identifying the problem—"the discrepancy between current and desired behavior," according to the family's point of view—Jennifer's mother and grandmother agreed to continue with the next step. They felt that it was appropriate to observe Jennifer's motor behaviors at home and to document her specific competencies and patterns of functioning. The consultant assisted in devising a plan for collecting this information. The data collection procedure, a simple checklist of specific motor behaviors, was one that Jennifer's family members felt they could handle in their situation because it would not entail a large amount of time to complete.

A second consultation session was scheduled to occur one week later. The information that the family members were to gather in regard to Jennifer's movement abilities would be used during this subsequent interview to identify specific goals and to design a plan for intervention, including direct and indirect physical therapy services.

In future consultation meetings, Jennifer's family and the consultant will build upon observation and problem-solving skills developed in earlier sessions. Further independence and enablement of the consultees (the family) will be facilitated through the consultative process.

• • •

Drawing from the consultation expertise of other professions will assist early intervention personnel in effectively acting as consultants. As consultants, early interventionists may indirectly deliver appropriate services to their clients—infants and toddlers with special needs. This goal is accomplished in consultation by building collaborative relationships with the consultees (families, day care providers, and other early interventionists).

Parents say that their major areas of need are for information and support,[15,16] both of which consultation readily provides in a less intrusive format. In addition, consultation is appropriate for families who desire early intervention services focusing primarily on child outcomes rather than on family support issues. Consultation, therefore, should be used and researched as a viable option in service delivery models to effectively and efficiently meet the needs of some infants and toddlers with special needs and their families.

REFERENCES

1. Gilkerson L, Hilliard A, Schrag E, Shonkoff P. Point of view: Commenting on P.L. 99-457. *Zero to Three.* 1987;7(3):13–17.

2. Institute of Medicine. Committee to Study the Role of Allied Health Personnel, William Richardson, Chairman. *Allied Health Services: Avoiding Crises.* Washington, DC: National Academy Press, 1989.

3. Meisels S, Harbin G, Modigliani K, Olson K. Formulating optimal state early childhood intervention policies. *Except Child.* 1988;55:159–165.

4. Yoder D, Coleman P, Gallagher J. *Allied Health Personnel: Meeting the Demands of Part H, Public Law 99-457.* Chapel Hill, NC: Carolina Institute for Child and Family Policy, 1990.

5. Campbell P. Preparing personnel to work in early intervention. In: Kaiser A, McWhorter C, eds. *Preparing Personnel To Work with Persons with Severe Disabilities.* Baltimore, MD: Paul H. Brookes, 1990.

6. Affleck G, Tennen H, Rowe J, Roscher B, Walker L. Effects of formal support on mothers; Adaptation to the hospital-to-home transition of high risk infants: The benefits and costs of helping. *Child Dev.* 1989;60:488–501.

7. Johnston K. Mental health consultation to day care providers: The San Francisco daycare consultants program. *Zero to Three.* 1990;10(3):7–10.

8. Brown D, Pryzwansky W, Schulte A. *Psychological Consultation: Introduction to Theory and Practice.* Boston: Allyn & Bacon, 1987.

9. Erchul W, Conoley C. Helpful theories to guide the counselor's practice of school-based consultation. *Elem School Guidance Counsel.* In press.

10. Dunst C, Trivette C, Deal A. *Enabling and Empowering Families.* Cambridge, Mass: Brookline Books, 1988.

11. Meisels S, Shonkoff J. *Handbook of Early Childhood Intervention.* New York: Cambridge University Press, 1990.

12. Bergan J. *Behavioral Consultation.* Columbus, OH: Charles E. Merrill, 1977.

13. Bailey D. Collaborative goal-setting with families: Resolving differences in values and priorities for services. *Top Early Child Spec Educ.* 1987;2:39–71.

14. Wright J, Granger R, Sameroff A. Parental acceptance and developmental handicap. In: Blacher J, ed. *Severely Handicapped Young Children and Their Families: Research in Review.* Orlando: Academic Press, 1983.

15. Bailey D, Blasco P, Simeonsson R. The structure and nature of family needs in early intervention. *J Early Intervent.* In press.

16. Summers J, Dell'Oliver C, Turnbull A, et al. Focusing in on the IFSP process: What are family and practitioner preferences? *Top Early Child Spec Educ.* In press.

Efficacy of therapeutic intervention intensity with infants and young children with cerebral palsy

Howard P. Parette, Jr., EdD
Assistant Professor
Center for Research on Teaching and
   Learning
University of Arkansas at Little Rock

Mary D. Hendricks, PhD
Assistant Professor
Department of Teacher Education
University of Arkansas at Little Rock
Little Rock, Arkansas

Stephen L. Rock, PhD
Director
Research and Educational Planning
   Center
College of Education
University of Nevada–Reno
Reno, Nevada

PHYSICAL THERAPY and occupational therapy are two of the most frequently employed means for the provision of early therapeutic intervention with children who have cerebral palsy[1-3] and are integral components of federally mandated services via Public Law 94-142, Education of All Handicapped Children Act of 1975, and Public Law 99-457, Education of the Handicapped Act, Amendments 1986. In an era when diminishing fiscal resources seem to be affecting service delivery systems with increasing intensity, school systems and other service providers will, of necessity, begin to examine more closely questions relating to therapeutic intervention effectiveness. Issues such as the efficacy of therapy with specific types of children, the forms of therapy that are most effective, and whether or not the effects of therapy are maintained over time will become critical in decision-making processes.[1,4] In a similar vein, the efficacy of alternative forms of therapeutic intervention service delivery, such as family-focused interventions[5-8] and parent/child groups,[9] will have to be investigated.

The effects of therapeutic intervention strategies have been far from definitive.[2,8,10-12] This has placed considerable pressures on service providers and the scientific community to adhere to rigorous research approaches to determine the efficacy of various intervention approaches with infants and young children who have cerebral palsy. Of particular importance are the contributory effects of specific subject and treatment variables on therapeutic intervention outcomes.[2,10,13,14] Studies have suggested that subject variables such as mental competence,[15-17] age,[18,19] type of cerebral palsy,[20,21] emotional disturbance,[12,22] and degree of involvement[14,23] (also: Parette HP, Hourcade JJ. April 1990. Unpublished data) interact to affect children's responses to the interventions. Similarly, treatment variables such as type of intervention[8,19] have also been reported to have an impact upon children's responses to physical therapy and occupational therapy. One treatment variable that has received relatively little attention in the professional habilitation literature is intensity of treatment.

Intensity and frequency of therapeutic intervention services are terms often used interchangeably in research on outcomes of occupational therapy and physical therapy strategies with children who have cerebral palsy. Earlier reports have typically reflected the prevailing position taken by occupational therapists and physical therapists that treatment provided to children is highly individualized and depends on the child and his or her individual needs.[24,25] For example, Phelps[26] stated that daily 1-hour treatment sessions for 6 weeks to 3 months should produce results in the child if any are to be obtained. Conversely, Crothers and Paine[27] suggested that rigid, prolonged, and closely supervised therapy is not always necessary but does have its place for some children.

Piper et al[3] found that high-risk infants receiving physical therapy failed to perform better than a control group of such children. These researchers suggested that their therapeutic intervention (ie, weekly 1-hour sessions) may have been too infrequent to effect positive outcomes. Previous studies conducted with culturally disadvantaged children have also implied that daily intensive intervention is required to derive positive outcomes,[28,29] though comparison groups of children not receiving therapeutic intervention were not included in such studies. Thus, it would seem that intensity of treatment, in a general sense, assumes dual dimensions of *frequency* and *duration*, which are inextricably interwoven in ways that are little understood. This lack of understanding is also reflected in the wide variability of how therapists view the manner in which intensity of treatment should be applied to children. Unfortunately, only three articles have addressed the issue of intensity of treatment, two of which failed to include children having cerebral palsy,[1,30] while the other categorized previous studies by measuring the trustworthiness of therapy efficacy reported.[31]

Lacking both empirical and theoretical structures for establishing treatment levels for children with cerebral palsy, professionals often have little choice but to rely on custom and intuition in making decisions.[1,25] In public school settings, some children may be scheduled to receive therapeutic intervention intermittently, such as once weekly, while others are treated on a daily basis but only for a short duration of time, such as 6 weeks. Public school officials who are charged with the responsibility of making decisions regarding the allocation of scarce resources are becoming concerned about how services such as physical therapy and occupational therapy should be provided under PL 94-142.[32,33] Similarly PL 99-457 specifies that the public schools are the payers of last resort for early intervention services, such as occupational and physical therapy for children from birth to 2 years,[34] placing even greater importance on justifications for the frequency of therapeutic regimens provided to this population.

DESCRIPTION OF THE STUDY

In order to address the need for a better understanding of intensity of treatment, a comprehensive *Index Medicus* and computer search of the therapeutic intervention effectiveness literature published between 1960 and 1989 was conducted. Intensity was defined as occupational therapy or physical therapy that was reported in the context of either frequency or duration of intervention. Duration included both the length of the therapy session and the duration of the intervention study. Included in the review were reports of children with a diagnosis of cerebral palsy, who were 5 years or less in age at the time that therapy was initiated. Reports describing only a single child were not considered, though numerous case studies relating to therapeutic intervention effectiveness have been published. Studies were classified in the following manner:

- ex post facto studies were categorized as no control group or descriptive;
- studies with two or more experimental groups with no control were categorized as contrast; and
- studies that employed control group methodology (both with and without random assignment) were categorized as control group.

Additionally, outcome measures were examined across studies, with an emphasis upon whether therapy intensity was reported to affect children's responses to treatment or whether a relationship was indicated by the data. Finally, studies were examined for suggestions relating to alternative forms of therapy such as therapist-supervised or parent-implemented intervention.

FINDINGS

A review of the literature generated 13 studies that met the categories described previously. A summary of these findings is presented in the Appendix (at end of article following commentaries).

Sample characteristics

As earlier reports have noted,[10,35,36] criteria for inclusion of subjects in studies that examined therapeutic intervention effectiveness have been far from rigid. Samples of infants and young children with various types of cerebral palsy have typically been drawn from only a limited geographic locale or have drawn from children being served at a particular center or facility.

Descriptive studies

Four studies were categorized as descriptive studies. The number of children in the treatment groups evidenced a wide range, with groups as small as three[37] and as large as 114[20] being reported. Those studies that have employed larger groups of children tend to reflect greater heterogeneity of age ranges.[15,20,38]

Contrast studies

Only six studies used a contrast or comparison group research design. Of these studies, sample sizes ranged from 12 children[19] to 48[2] to 194.[39] In all but one of these studies,[40] the types of cerebral palsy under consideration were described.

Control studies

Three studies were control studies. Characteristically, they used smaller groups of children. Parette[41] described the progress of 25 children, and Wright and Nicholson[12] described the progress of more than 40 children. One study investigated results in fewer than 30 children.[17] Of these three studies, only one provided detailed information regarding the types of cerebral palsy represented in the subjects.

Therapeutic intervention intensity

Descriptive studies

As shown in the appendix, the therapeutic intervention dimension of duration of therapy for groups of children varied from 9 months[37] to 4 years,[15] and the length of therapy sessions was generally unreported in descriptive studies, with the exception of Norton's study,[37] in which 1-hour treatment sessions were provided. The frequency of therapeutic intervention also varied markedly, ranging from once a year[38] to once a week[20] to daily sessions.[37]

Contrast studies

Four of the six contrast studies described specific treatment parameters relating to length and frequency of treatment. These parameters ranged from biweekly 1-hour sessions for 12 months[2] to 6-day-a-week, 1.5-hour sessions for 4 months.[42] Banham[40] specified only the duration of treatment, ranging from 12 to 22 months for respective treatment groups. One study provided only a mean and standard deviation for treatment duration.[39]

Control studies

The three control studies reported shorter periods of treatment. One reported treatment of 12 months[12] but failed to delineate the frequency of therapeutic intervention strategies provided or the length of therapy sessions. One[17] specified both the duration and frequency of intervention services; treatment reported in this study consisted of 30-minute sessions provided twice weekly for 5 months. The third study[41] reported "individualized" treatment sessions being provided to infants over a period of 6 months.

Instrumentation

Descriptive studies

Typically, these descriptive studies reported the use of nonstandardized assessment instruments, which addressed such aspects of functioning as fine motor skills[38] and general functional skills across several domains.[15,20] Only one study[37] employed a standardized evaluation instrument, though this study was severely limited in sample size.

Contrast studies

Three of the six contrast studies used standardized assessment instruments.[2,19,40] Two studies[8,42] reported the use of clinic-specific assessment instruments for documenting children's responses to therapeutic intervention. One study[39] employed Vojta screening and assessment procedures along with computed tomography scans to examine the severity of brain damage.

Control studies

The three control studies used two or more instruments to document responses to intervention.[12,17,41] One study[12] reported the use of a clinic-specific assessment instrument in combination with norm-referenced tests and clinical appraisals of physical and neurologic functioning. Another study[17] also described the use of a clinic-specific instrument along with a criterion-referenced instrument employing a well-defined system of coding and scoring performance and a noncalibrated set of guidelines developed by a professional organization. A third study[41] used a norm-referenced evaluation instrument in conjunction with a clinic-specific instrument.

Response to treatment and intensity impact

Descriptive studies

In all four descriptive studies reported in the appendix, children receiving therapeutic intervention demonstrated gains in motor functioning. Three studies suggested a relationship between the provision of intense regimens of therapy and positive motor outcomes: greater progress in those children receiving "adequate" treatment[20]; the attainment of higher developmental levels[37]; and a consistent relationship between number of treatments provided and greater motor progress.[38]

Contrast studies

The six studies employing a comparison group research design reported equivocal findings, with two of the studies conducted during the 1970s[40,42] indicating that treatment provided for a longer duration was critical for greater motor gains. A more recent study[2] reported that therapy provided more than twice monthly might not be as efficacious as other types of intervention.

Control studies

The implications of those studies that have used control group methodology are unclear. The authors of the earliest of these studies[12] commented that therapeutic gains subsequent to intense treatment generally are evidenced in nonmotoric areas, though they never addressed the issue of treatment intensity. One study[17] reported that less intense therapy, or other alternatives, may be indicated for this population. Another study[41] suggested that motor milestones measured by standardized assessment instruments might be obscured through the provision of therapeutic intervention strategies, although more subtle changes such as improved quality of motor acts or movement patterns might be observed.

DISCUSSION

A review of the available literature offers some support for the efficacy of therapeutic intervention for infants and young children with cerebral palsy. However, it fails to reveal any consensus relating to the delineation of "intense therapeutic intervention." Further, it reiterates the ongoing need to examine therapeutic efficacy. With increasing attention being placed upon the implementation of PL 99-457 across the country, the effectiveness of related services such as occupational therapy and physical therapy in these and other children will be even more carefully scrutinized. For professionals who will increasingly be called upon to make decisions regarding which children should receive therapeutic intervention, an attempt to clarify the meaning of the variable of intensity/frequency becomes important, because high service levels for some children may mean that other children will receive little or no services.[1]

The review of the existing literature on data collection and analytical tools used in both physical therapy and occupational therapy suggests that inadequate measurement of children's responses to therapeutic intervention is prevalent.[14,43,44] Traditionally, most therapists have relied on semiobjective, anecdotal reports or simple outcome studies for their evaluation of therapeutic programs.[37] Sometimes, a potentially effective treatment strategy may be deemed to be ineffective because of improper behavior selection and definition, poor measurement strategies, or the failure to evaluate environmental factors.[43] Often, children's failure to respond positively to treatment is attributed to their lack of motivation[22] or to the degree of brain damage.[14] Instead of examining variables that relate to the therapist, the child, or the type of therapy provided, therapists many times resort to attributing lack of progress to the child's behavior or organic condition.[14,43]

In addition to case reports and subjective clinical evaluations, a large number of assessment procedures and instruments typically have been employed to study the effects of therapy in young children who have cerebral palsy. Strategies employed that are readily identifiable in the literature include functional inventories and evaluations of activities of daily living,[15,45] skill tests,[46] motor ability tests,[8,47,48] developmental profiles,[49] and pattern analysis charts.[50]

In any given program serving children who have cerebral palsy, it is often unclear as to how decisions are made regarding the intensity of therapy.[51] Of particular concern is the growing impetus toward more creative programming options for the provision of needed related services to infants and young children with cerebral palsy. This has important implications for public school systems from a fiscal ethics perspective (ie, decisions on how resources are to be allocated for related services under PL 94-142 and PL 99-457). Piper[31] suggested that physical therapy must be provided a minimum of twice weekly to be efficacious in promoting motor milestone attainment. Barnett[32] has noted that the resources needed to adequately provide such services to all handicapped children under existing legislation are inadequate, thus suggesting the need for states to develop alternative models of service delivery that might potentially be based on cost, child progress, or other long-term benefits. Greater attention might be focused on alternative approaches to treatment, such as therapist-supervised, parent-implemented therapy, which could be provided at less expense on a more frequent basis to those children in need of services.

As the habilitation professions continue to examine the effectiveness of therapeutic intervention for children with cerebral palsy, alternatives to traditional intervention are likely to emerge. The demand for accountability in all fields of intervention has been perceived as a call for "developmental physical and occupational therapists to provide objective, systematic documentation of the results of our treatment efforts."[52(p30)] Professionals must continue to investigate the process of evaluating treatment effectiveness; defining the parameters of treatment is necessary if firm conclusions are to be made about what works and how much treatment is necessary.[53] The therapeutic intervention literature is replete with calls that greater attention be given to such treatment parameters as intelligence, degree and type of involvement, age at entry into program, emotional disturbance, and type of treatment approach employed. The efficacy of specific treatment methodologies for specific children will remain clouded by uncertainty if occupational therapists and physical therapists do not achieve consensus regarding the variables that guide and direct their research. "Intensity" is a critical variable requiring clarification and careful delineation if the implications of the researcher's treatment effects are to be fully realized.

• • •

A newly emerging database is being reflected in the field of early intervention research. Heightened levels of sophistication are consistently demonstrated in reported studies, characterized by the use of experimental designs that minimize threats to internal validity, careful documentation of procedures and outcomes, and approaches that incorporate theories of general child development.[54] Physical and occupational therapy research is similarly affected as calls for accountability become increasingly evident in the professional literature.[10,11] With such changes transpiring both within these disciplines and in the systems that employ them, changes may be anticipated with regard to how the intensity of therapeutic intervention is viewed and applied.

REFERENCES

1. Jenkins JR, Sells CJ. Physical and occupational therapy: Effects related to treatment, frequency, and motor delay. *J Learn Disab.* 1984;17:89–95.

2. Palmer FB, Shapiro BK, Wachtel RC, et al. The effects of physical therapy on cerebral palsy. *N Engl J Med.* 1988;318:803–808.

3. Piper MC, Kunos VI, Willis DM, Mazer BL, Ramsay M, Silver KM. Early physical therapy effects on the high-risk infant: A randomized controlled trial. *Pediatrics.* 1986;78:216–224.

4. Goodman M, Rothberg AD, Houston-McMillan JE, Cooper PA, Cartwright JE, Ven der Velde MA. Effect of early neurodevelopmental therapy in normal and at-risk survivors of neonatal intensive care. *Lancet.* 1985;2:1327–1331.

5. Ottenbacher K, Petersen P. The efficacy of early intervention programs for children with organic impairment: A quantitative review. *Eval Program Plann.* 1985;8:135–146.

6. Parette HP, Hourcade JJ. Parental participation in early therapeutic intervention programs for young children with cerebral palsy: An unresolved dilemma. *Rehabil Lit.* 1985;46:2–7.

7. Rainforth B, Salisbury CL. Functional home programs: A model for therapists. *Top Early Child Spec Educ.* 1988;7:33–45.

8. Scherzer AL, Mike V, Ilson J. Physical therapy as a determinant of change in the cerebral palsied infant. *Pediatrics.* 1976;58:47–52.

9. Tyler NB, Chandler LS. The developmental therapists: The occupational therapist and physical therapist. In: Allen KE, Holm VA, Schiefelbusch RL, eds. *Early Intervention: A Team Approach.* Baltimore: University Park Press, 1978.

10. Parette HP, Hourcade JJ. A review of therapeutic intervention research on gross and fine motor progress in young children with cerebral palsy. *Am J Occup Ther.* 1984; 38:462–468.

11. Tirosh E, Rabino S. Physiotherapy for children with cerebral palsy. *Am J Dis Child.* 1989;143:552–555.

12. Wright T, Nicholson J. Physiotherapy for the spastic child: An evaluation. *Dev Med Child Neurol.* 1973;15:146–163.

13. Gonella C. Designs for clinical research. *Phys Ther.* 1973;53:1276–1283.

14. Martin JE, Epstein LH. Evaluating treatment effectiveness in cerebral palsy. *Phys Ther.* 1976;56:285–294.

15. Footh WK, Kogan KL. Measuring the effectiveness of physical therapy in the treatment of cerebral palsy. *J Am Phys Ther Assoc.* 1963;43:867–873.
16. Parette HP, Hourcade JJ. How effective are physiotherapeutic programmes with young mentally retarded children who have cerebral palsy? *J Ment Defic Res.* 1984;28:167–175.
17. Sommerfeld D, Fraser BA, Hensinger RN, Beresford CV. Evaluation of physical therapy service for severely mentally impaired students with cerebral palsy. *Phys Ther.* 1981;61:338–344.
18. Brandt S, Lonstrup H, Marner T, Rump KJ, Selman P, Schack LK. Prevention of cerebral palsy in motor-risk infants by treatment ad modum Vojta. *Acta Paediatr Scand.* 1980;69:283–286.
19. Carlsen PN. Comparison of two occupational therapy approaches for treating the young cerebral palsied child. *Am J Occup Ther.* 1975;29:267–272.
20. Karlsson B, Nauman B, Gardestrom L. Results of physical treatment in cerebral palsy. *Cerebral Palsy Bull.* 1960;2:278–285.
21. Zuck FN, Johnson MK. The progress of cerebral palsy patients under in-patient circumstances. In: American Academy of Orthopaedic Surgeons, eds. *Instructional Course Lectures*, vol 9. Ann Arbor, MI: J. W. Edwards, 1952.
22. Hourcade JJ, Parette HP Jr. Cerebral palsy and emotional disturbance: A review and implications. *J Rehabil.* 1984;50:55–60.
23. D'Avignon MD, Noren L, Arman T. Early physiotherapy ad modum Vojta or Bobath in infants with suspected neuromotor disturbances. *Neuropediatrics.* 1981;12:232–241.
24. Levitt S. *Treatment of Cerebral Palsy and Motor Delay.* Oxford: Blackwell, 1977.
25. Denhoff E, Robinault IP. *Cerebral Palsy and Related Disorders: A Developmental Approach to Dysfunction.* New York: McGraw-Hill, 1960.
26. Phelps W. The cerebral palsy problem. *Postgrad Med.* 1950;7:206–209.
27. Crothers B, Paine RS. *The Natural History of Cerebral Palsy.* Cambridge, MA: Harvard University Press, 1959.
28. Heber R, Garber H. The Milwaukee project: A study of the use of family intervention to parent cultural-familial retardation. In: Friedlander B, Sterritt G, Kirk G, eds. *Exceptional Infant. Assessment and Intervention.* New York: Brunner/Mazel, 1975.
29. Ramey C, Smith BJ. Assessing the intellectual consequences of early intervention with high-risk infants. *Am J Ment Defic.* 1976;81:318–324.
30. Jenkins JR, Sells CJ, Brady D, et al. Effects of occupational and physical therapy in a school program. *Phys Occup Ther Pediatr.* 1982;4:19–29.
31. Piper MC. Efficacy of physical therapy: Rate of motor development in children with cerebral palsy. *Pediatr Phys Ther.* 1990;2:126–130.
32. Barnett WS. The economics of preschool special education under Public Law 99-457. *Top Early Child Spec Educ.* 1988;8:12–23.
33. Smith BJ, Strain PS. Early childhood special education in the next decade: Implementing and expanding P.L. 99-457. *Top Early Child Spec Educ.* 1988;8:37–47.
34. Fox HB, Freedman SA, Klepper SA, Klepper BR. Financing programs for young children with handicaps. In: Gallagher JJ, Trohanis PL, Clifford RM, eds. *Policy Implementation & P.L. 99-457. Planning for Young Children with Special Needs.* Baltimore: Paul H. Brookes, 1989.
35. Dunst CJ, Rheingrover RM. An analysis of the efficacy of infant intervention programs with organically handicapped children. *Eval Prog Plann.* 1981; 4:287–323.
36. Simeonsson RJ, Cooper DH, Scheiner AP. A review and analysis of the effectiveness of early intervention programs. *Pediatrics.* 1982;69:635–641 .
37. Norton Y. Neurodevelopment and sensory integration for the profoundly retarded multiply handicapped child. *Am J Occup Ther.* 1975;29:93–100.

38. Tyler NB, Kogan KL. Measuring effectiveness of occupational therapy. *Am J Occup Ther.* 1965;19:8–13.

39. Kanda T, Yuge M, Yamori Y, Suzuki J, Fukase H. Early physiotherapy in the treatment of spastic diplegia. *Dev Med Child Neurol.* 1984;26:438–444.

40. Banham KM. Progress in motor development of retarded cerebral palsied infants. *Rehabil Lit.* 1976; 37:13–14.

41. Parette HP. *The Relationship of Specific Variables to Motoric Gains in Infants Who Have Cerebral Palsy or Motor Delay: A Comparative Treatment Study.* Tuscaloosa, AL: University of Alabama; 1982. Dissertation.

42. Abdel-Salam E, Maraghi S, Tawfik M. Evaluation of physical therapy techniques in the management of cerebral palsy. *J Egypt Med Assoc.* 1978;61:531–541.

43. Carr BS, Williams M. Analysis of therapeutic techniques through use of the standard behavior chart. Implications for physical therapy. *Phys Ther.* 1982;52:177–183.

44. Whitney PL. Measurement for curriculum building for multiply handicapped children. *Phys Ther.* 1978; 58:415–420.

45. Ingram AJ, Withers E, Spelt E. Role of intensive physical and occupational therapy in the treatment of cerebral palsy: Testing and results. *Arch Phys Med Rehab.* 1959;40:429–438.

46. Crosland JH. The assessment of results in the conservative treatment of cerebral palsy. *Arch Dis Child.* 1951;26:92–95.

47. Johnson MK, Zuck FN, Wingate K. The motor age test: Measurement of motor handicaps in children with neuromuscular disorders such as cerebral palsy. *J Bone Joint Surg [Am].* 1951;33:698–707.

48. Zausmer E, Tower G. A quotient for the evaluation of motor development. *J Am Phys Ther Assoc.* 1966;46:725–728.

49. Doman GJ, Delacato CH, Doman RJ. *The Doman-Delacato Developmental Mobility Scale.* Philadelphia: The Rehabilitation Center, 1960.

50. Milani-Comparetti A, Gidoni EA. Pattern analysis of motor development and its disorders. *Dev Med Child Neurol.* 1967;9:625–630.

51. Haley SM. Patterns of physical and occupational therapy implementation in early motor intervention. *Top Early Child Spec Educ.* 1988;7:46–63.

52. Harris SR. Early intervention: Does developmental therapy make a difference? *Top Early Child Spec Educ.* 1988;7:20–32.

53. Bailey DB, Simeonsson RJ. Design issues in family impact evaluation. In: Bickman L, Weatherford DL, eds. *Evaluating Early Intervention Programs for Severely Handicapped Children and Their Families.* Austin, TX: Pro-Ed, 1986.

54. Guralnick MJ. Recent developments in early intervention efficacy research: Implications for family involvement in P.L. 99-457. *Top Early Child Spec Educ.* 1989;9:1–17.

Editor's note: *The previous article by Parette, Hendricks, and Rock raised several important issues regarding the cost effectiveness of certain interventions. We asked several experts in the fields of occupational therapy and physical therapy to respond. We hope you will find all three contributions provocative.*

Commentary

Barbara Hanft, OTR/L, MA, FAOTA
Consultant and Trainer
Silver Spring, Maryland

Charlotte Brasic Royeen, OTR, PhD, FAOTA
Research and Therapy Services
Great Falls, Virginia

We welcome the opportunity to comment upon the discussion presented by Parette, Hendricks, and Rock that the intensity (ie, frequency and duration) of therapy is an important issue to study. We believe, however, that the authors' discussion of intensity is too narrow. How much is enough therapy for children with cerebral palsy is a question that can only be considered in the context of each child's profile of abilities and delays, the service setting, and who is providing the care. Before proceeding, however, we wish to discuss three related but distinctly different terms that we have paraphrased from a noteworthy discussion on research by Pless.[1] The terms are efficacy, effectiveness, and efficiency.

- Efficacy refers to documenting that an intervention is more beneficial than it is harmful.
- Effectiveness refers to documenting that an efficacious intervention can be realistically applied to a target population.
- Efficiency refers to documenting the effectiveness of an intervention with the least expenditures of time, personnel, and money.

According to these definitions, we would argue that the body of research related to therapeutic intervention with infants and young children clearly shows it to be efficacious but not efficient (ie, other interventions may be less expensive and as effective). Parette, Hendricks, and Rock may really be calling for more studies of efficiency rather than efficacy.

UNIDIMENSIONAL VS MULTIDIMENSIONAL

Parette et al asked, "What is the efficacy of therapeutic intervention intensity with infants and young children with cerebral palsy?" This is an important question, but it reflects a unidimensional view that may be too simplistic. Instead, we believe a multidimensional view is required when evaluating the efficiency of services to any population. A multidimensional view of the efficiency of therapeutic intensity with infants and young children with cerebral palsy would have to address (and not just as a limitation) myriad factors in relationship to each other, as follows[2]:

- Entry criteria (who will benefit?).
- What is the intervention?

- What is the frequency of intervention?
- What is the duration of intervention?
- Who provides the intervention (therapist, aide, family member, or combination thereof)?
- Where is the intervention provided?
- What are the expected outcomes of intervention?
- Exit criteria (will continued intervention yield beneficial results?).

PHASES OF RESEARCH

A second issue we wish to address relates to how empirical data on intervention research is developed over time. By discounting all single subject research regarding the efficacy of therapeutic intensity, Parette, Hendricks, and Rock miss an important body of knowledge. We would argue that single case studies provide an opportunity to gather data important to identifying parameters and testing the effectiveness of intervention prior to launching large clinical trials. One of the premier medical journals in the country, the *New England Journal of Medicine*, publishes a case study in each edition.

Gonella described four phases of knowledge development related to clinical trial research, which are instrumental for understanding the importance of single subject research, as well as other nonexperimental research, such as descriptive correlational and intervention studies.[3] The four phases in Table 1 represent the big picture regarding the development of a body of knowledge for a particular intervention.

Table 1 identifies a hierarchical arrangement, with phase 4 research dependent upon information obtained in previous phases. Though single subject research can be executed to address factors related to phases 3 and 4, it is most often employed when developing a database (phases 1 and 2). A rush to execute clinical trials in phase 4, without adequate preparation in the previous phases, assures contradictory and confounded comparative studies.

Table 1. Four phases of knowledge development related to clinical trial research

Research phase	Purpose
Phase 1	Identify parameters of interest.
Phase 2	Describe the effectiveness of the intervention with a number of patients.
Phase 3	Estimate the predictability or reliability of the intervention across patients.
Phase 4	Execute comparative clinical trials.

DIFFERENCES IN CLINICAL PRACTICE

Parette, Hendricks, and Rock treat occupational and physical therapy as though they were interchangeable interventions. While desired outcomes may be similar (ie, that children function at age appropriate levels) it is a mistake not to acknowledge differences in treatment objectives and modalities of each discipline. The modality, or specific intervention, chosen by each professional will influence the intensity of treatment. Each profession has diverse treatment approaches that cannot be generically grouped together. Moreover, data from "therapy" studies that include both physical and occupational therapy interventions should also not be grouped together without carefully analyzing the specific services provided. Teaching a child to button his or her shirt vs improving postural stability or eye-hand coordination requires differing amounts of therapist involvement. Working through other professionals or parents vs providing "hands-on" therapy to reach the desired outcome is another variable that will influence the intensity of services.

The question of intensity of services, then, is appropriate to raise *only* within a specific treatment context related to the therapist's professional orientation and accepted standards for best practice. Asking how often therapy should be offered without identifying the desired outcomes is similar to asking what the best age or height is—for what purpose? Research regarding the intensity of therapy is multidimensional and must be connected to the purpose for therapy.

SETTING AND INTENSITY

We agree with Parette et al that an important rationale for looking at the intensity of therapy is the interest of school administrators in implementing Public Law 94-142 and Public Law 99-457. However, these laws, their accompanying regulations, and related judicial decisions define how and when therapy can be provided.

Under PL 94-142, physical and occupational therapy can be provided *only as related services* to help a child benefit from special education.[4] In contrast, PL 99-457 identifies physical and occupational therapy as *primary* services (not tied to special education) that can be offered to assist infants and toddlers with disabilities and their family members.[5] Therefore, occupational or physical therapy provided to a preschool child with cerebral palsy in the school system must be educationally relevant. That same child could receive very different services from a physical or occupational therapist in a private clinic or medical setting.

Therefore, any study addressing the intensity of therapy for children must also look at the context or setting in which the therapy is provided. Again, the question of intensity of services is a multidimensional question, that is, how much therapy is needed to reach the desired outcome for a child with a specific condition and ability profile?

DIAGNOSIS AND INTENSITY

By selecting a diagnostic category for studying the intensity of services, Parette et al imposed an arbitrary classification on their analysis. Therapists do not treat cerebral palsy; they treat the limitations in function and mobility accompanying the condition. By reviewing studies whose subjects were children with cerebral palsy, Parette, Hendricks, and Rock imply, incorrectly, that there is a yet-undetermined "correct" number of hours of therapy to provide. Obviously, children with cerebral palsy demonstrate a very wide continuum of abilities and delays.

We agree that grouping children by diagnosis may help differentiate the outcome of therapy for children who have cerebral palsy vs a different condition such as closed head trauma. However, when considering the question of how much therapy to provide, it is equally important to look at the degree of involvement, the profile of the child's functional abilities and limitations, and the desired outcome of intervention.

RECOMMENDATIONS

In reviewing the literature regarding the intensity of therapy for young children with cerebral palsy, Parette, Hendricks, and Rock have raised an important issue for clinicians and researchers to consider. We believe it is vital for future research to address this issue in a multidimensional context, as it relates to the real world in which services are provided for children. Few insights have been provided regarding the functional relationship between methodology and desired outcomes in early intervention programs.[6] It is simply not helpful to ask how often physical or occupational therapy should be provided without framing the questions within a multidimensional framework that address who needs therapy, for what reason, and who will provide it in what setting.

REFERENCES

1. Pless IB. On doubting and certainty. *Pediatrics.* 1976;58:7–9.
2. Olney SJ. Efficacy of movement in cerebral palsy. *Pediatr Phys Ther.* 1990;145–154.
3. Gonella C. Designs for clinical research. *Phys Ther.* 1973;53:1276–1283.
4. Hanft BE. The changing environment for early intervention services: Implications for practice. *Am J Occup Ther.* 1988;42:724–731.
5. Royeen CB, ed. Occupational therapy in the schools. *Am J Occup Ther.* 1988;42:697–750.
6. Dunst C, Snyder S. A critique of the Utah State University early intervention programs with organically handicapped children. *Except Child.* 1986;53:269–276.

Commentary

Susan R. Harris, PT, PhD, FAPT
Associate Professor
School of Rehabilitation Medicine
University of British Columbia
Vancouver, BC, Canada

While I concur with the desire of Parette, Hendricks, and Rock to examine the effects of therapeutic treatment intensity for young children with cerebral palsy, I do not feel that their extensive review of the early intervention efficacy literature adds much to our understanding of the central question: "Is more therapy better than less?" Although the authors are correct in reporting that the issue of treatment intensity has not been addressed in the research literature concerning young children with cerebral palsy, the study conducted by Jenkins and colleagues[1,2] during the early 1980s involving preschoolers with motor delays deserves more than the passing comment that was received in this review. Since the two articles based on this study are the *only* ones in the therapeutic intervention literature to address the topic of treatment intensity, they warrant further description.

RESEARCH ON TREATMENT INTENSITY

The earlier article by Jenkins and colleagues[1] examined the effects of different intensities of developmental therapy on the gross motor and fine motor performance of 45 preschool and schoolaged children with significant motor delays, as indicated by scores on the pediatric screening tool (PST).[3] The children were stratified according to their scores on the PST and then randomly assigned to one of three groups. The developmental therapy intervention was described as a combination of procedures derived from sensory integration and neurodevelopmental treatment (NDT). Children in the first group received treatment three times a week, children in the second group received treatment once a week, and children in the third group served as a no-treatment control. Treatment sessions were 40 minutes in duration and took place over a 15-week period. All of the children were pre- and posttested on the gross motor and fine motor portions of the Peabody Developmental Motor Scales (PDMS)[4] and on a seven-item scale measuring quality and maturity of postural reactions.

Children in the two treatment groups made significantly greater gains on the PDMS gross motor scores than children in the control group. However, there was no significant difference in gains between the group that received treatment three times a week when compared to the once-weekly treatment group. On the fine motor portion of the PDMS, the children in the two treatment groups made greater gains than the children in the control group, but the differences were not statistically significant. All three groups showed significant improvements on the postural reactions scale, but there were no between-group differences in gain scores. In their discussion of these results, the authors made the following comments:

> One of the more remarkable findings in this research relates to frequency and quantity of treatment. On the PDMS gross motor scale there was evidence of a significant therapy effect, but this effect did not vary with the quantity of therapy provided. Children who received therapy one time a week did as well as those who received three times that amount.[1(p27)]

In a follow-up article elaborating on this research, Jenkins and Sells[2] examined the possibility of different effects of the therapy on children at high and low need for therapy based on their scores on the PST and the PDMS pretest. Children who were more delayed initially based on PDMS developmental motor quotients and who received treatment made large and significant gains on the gross motor scale, whereas the less-delayed children made the same amount of gain regardless of whether or not they received therapy. The authors concluded. "Thus, by determining a motor quotient based on PDMS pretest, it was possible to predict which students would benefit from therapy."[2(p92)] There were no differential effects, however, on PDMS fine motor scores. In the final sentence of this important article, published in 1984, the authors made a plea for replication of this study. However, as Parette and colleagues have noted, no such replications have been published in the intervening 7 years.

CONSENSUS STATEMENTS ON TREATMENT INTENSITY

In the proceedings of a recent consensus conference examining the efficacy of physical therapy in the management of cerebral palsy, Piper[5] examined the issue of treatment intensity/frequency by carefully and systematically summarizing results of 14 studies that had evaluated the effects of physical therapy on promoting the rate of motor development for children with cerebral palsy. Based on the three studies that had employed randomized trials and had demonstrated clear-cut results,[6-8] Piper concluded that "Physical therapy, in order to be efficacious in promoting motor milestone attainment, must be offered a minimum of two times a week."[5(p129)] It is important to note, however, that the final consensus statements summarizing the results of this landmark conference decried the use of motor milestone acquisition as the sole or primary outcome measure in most previous effficacy studies, to the exclusion of more important and more relevant treatment outcomes such as prevention of contractures and deformities; improvements in posture, functional independence, family coping and physical management of the child; and cost/benefit analyses.[9]

DIRECTIONS FOR FUTURE RESEARCH

The issue of *optimal* treatment intensity for infants and young children with cerebral palsy remains to be addressed. Previous studies on children with cerebral palsy[6-8] have suggested that twice-weekly therapy is needed to effect attainment of motor milestones,[5] but none of these studies was specifically directed at examining the effects of different treatment intensities. No studies have been published that have addressed systematically the effects of varying intensities of therapy on outcomes, such as postural control, functional motor skills, and family adaptations for the child with cerebral palsy.

In spite of pleas by Jenkins and colleagues[1,2] for replication of their study examining the effects of treatment intensity on motor milestone attainment and postural responses in young children with motor delays, no replications have been published. In light of their finding that therapy conducted three times a week was no more efficacious than that conducted once a week, it would seem entirely ethical to partially replicate their design using a sample of young children with cerebral palsy. Rather than including a no-treatment control group, the third group could be a contrast group, that would receive a developmental stimulation program similar to the Learningames curriculum[10] that was used by Palmer and colleagues.[7]

While the authors of *this* review article are to be commended for raising the important issue of the relationship of treatment intensity to therapeutic outcome, their article falls short in describing and elucidating the existing research on this topic. It is hoped that this commentary will provide additional food for thought on this important topic and will prompt readers to consider the need for replications of previous studies examining the issue of treatment intensity.

Addendum: Subsequent to the submission of this commentary, an article[11] was published that examined the issue of treatment intensity for young children with cerebral palsy. Although the independent and dependent variables were somewhat different than those examined by Jenkins and colleagues,[1,2] the results were surprisingly similar in that the group that received three times as much NDT did not do significantly better than the group that received less intensive treatment. Readers are advised to review this important study and evaluate its implications concerning treatment intensity.

REFERENCES

1. Jenkins JR, Sells CJ, Brady D, Down J, Moore B, Carman P, et al. Effects of developmental therapy on motor impaired children. *Phys Occup Ther Pediatr.* 1982;2(4):19–28.
2. Jenkins JR, Sells CJ. Physical and occupational therapy: Effects related to treatment, frequency, and motor delay. *J Learn Disabil.* 1984; 17:89–95.

3. Taylor D, Christopher M, Freshman S. *Pediatric Screening: A Tool for Occupational and Physical Therapists*. Seattle: University of Washington Health Sciences Learning Resources Center, 1978.

4. Folio R, DuBose RF. *Peabody Developmental Motor Scales*. Revised experimental edition. IMRID Behav Res Mon No. 25. Nashville, Tenn: George Peabody College for Teachers, 1974.

5. Piper MC. Efficacy of physical therapy: Rate of motor development in children with cerebral palsy. *Pediatr Phys Ther.* 1990;2:126–130.

6. Carlsen P. Comparison of two occupational therapy approaches for treating the young cerebral-palsied child. *Am J Occup Ther.* 1975;29:267–272.

7. Palmer FB, Shapiro BK, Wachtel RC, Allen MC, Hiller JE, Harryman SE, et al. The effects of physical therapy on cerebral palsy: A controlled trial in infants with spastic diplegia. *N Engl J Med.* 1988;318:803–808.

8. Scherzer AL, Mike V, Ilson J. Physical therapy as a determinant of change in the cerebral palsied infant. *Pediatrics.* 1976;58:47–52.

9. Campbell SK. Consensus statements. In: Campbell SK, ed. Proceedings of the Consensus Conference on the Efficacy of Physical Therapy in the Management of Cerebral Palsy. *Pediatr Phys Ther.* 1990;2:175–176.

10. Sparling J, Lewis I. *Learningames for the First Three Years*. New York: Walker, 1979.

11. Law M, Cadman D, Rosenbaum P, Walter S, Russell D, DeMateo C. Neurodevelopmental therapy and upper-extremity inhibitive casting for children with cerebral palsy. *Dev Med Child Neurol* 1991;33:379–387.

Appendix

Description of studies relating to intensity of therapeutic intervention for infants and young children who have cerebral palsy

Study	Sample characteristics	Intensity of intervention program	Instrumentation	Response to treatment and intensity impact
Descriptive studies				
Karlsson, Nauman, & Gardestrom[20]	114 children ages birth–>10 yrs.; type of cp: 42 (hemipegia), 21 (paraplegia), 18 (tetraplegia), 13 (athetosis), 8 (ataxia), 12 (mixed); 24 children in birth–2 yr. age group, of which 21% had tetraplegia & 29% were of lowest functional levels; 40 children in 3–6 yr. age group, with 18% having tetraplegia and 48% being of lowest functional capacity; 33 children in 7–10 yr. age group, with 12% having tetraplegia and 39% being of lowest functional capacity; 17 children in >10 yr. age group, with 12% having tetraplegia and 35% being of the lowest functional level	Physical therapy 1–3 times weekly in clinic or in home for at least 3 yrs.	Minear (1956) Classification System; Hartwell Motor Age Test	Motor performance improved in 54% of the subjects, with the greatest progress being demonstrated in children who received treatment deemed to be "adequate," had a diagnosis of athetosis and ataxia, were between 1–2 yrs. of age, and had higher IQs.

Study	Sample characteristics	Intensity of intervention program	Instrumentation	Response to treatment and intensity impact
Footh, Kogan[15]	73 children, ages 10–63 mo. (with children being in program >1 yr. being counted more than once): <3 yrs. (60), 3–4 yrs. (30), 5–6 yrs. (12); spastic diplegia (46), athetosis (35), spastic hemiplegia (26), mixed (12)	Unspecified individualized treatment provided over 4-yr. period (range, 1 time per mo.—daily therapy)	Preschool Functional Activity Test	Therapy found to be more advantageous for younger children (<3 yrs.); children with diplegia or athetosis have better motoric gain prognosis than hemiplegics; therapy unrelated to motor gains; suggested the importance of parental role in the provision of therapy
Tyler, Kogan[18]	77 children, ages 10–63 mos. half of whom were mentally retarded; for 137 testing sessions (no more than 3 tests on each child), diagnoses included spastic diplegia (59); athetosis (32); spastic hemiplegia (29); and mixed (17)	Unspecified individualized treatment provided over 3-yr. period (range, 1 time per yr.–daily therapy)	Children's Hand Skills Survey	Relationship of motor improvement found to exist with all study variables (amount of therapy, initial score, therapy history, diagnosis, IQ, and age): consistent relationship between no. of treatments given and achievement of higher gains; children with milder upper extremity involvement might benefit from an increased no. of sessions
Norton[37]	3 profoundly retarded children, 3–4 yrs. of age; diagnoses included: diffuse brain damage: mixed cerebral palsy; and cerebral atrophy, microcephaly, and hydrocephaly	Home program applied by therapist-trained mothers, 1 hr. per day for 9 mos.	Milani-Comparetti & Gidoni developmental examination	Treatment resulted in the attainment of higher developmental levels (postural, emotional, perceptual, cognitive); suggested that intensity of treatment can affect the maturation level of the central nervous system in multihandicapped, retarded children who have experienced sensory integration

Study	Sample characteristics	Intensity of intervention program	Instrumentation	Response to treatment and intensity impact
Contrast studies Carlsen[19]	Two groups of 6 children, ages 1–5 yrs., matched by CA, MA, and diagnosis: spasticity (8); athetoid (3); mixed (1);	Each child received 1-hr. sessions twice weekly for 6 wks.	Bayley Mental and Motor scales; DDST	Children receiving facilitation approach demonstrated more significant improvement than children receiving functional approach
Scherzer, Mike, Ilson[8]	22 children <18 mos. of age; athetosis (11), spasticity (6), mixed (2), ataxia (1), MR (1), brain damage (1)	14 children assigned to experimental group, 8 assigned to contrast group; therapy was provided twice weekly up to the age of 2 yrs. for both groups (mean = 12 mo. treatment using neurophysiologic PT and parent-provided therapy for experimental group; mean = 11 mo. treatment using passive range of motion exercises for control group)	Motor Development Evaluation Form	Superior gains demonstrated by treated group on motor status, social management, and home management by parents; greatest changes found to be inversely related to age at entry into study, and gains more often associated with least treatment time; suggested that other modalities of stimulation should be given greater emphasis during early years
Banham[40]	60 retarded children, mean age = 33 mos., mean IQ = 53; 11 nonretarded children, mean age = 21 mos., mean IQ = 100	41 retarded children provided with home program for 12 mos.; 19 retarded children provided with surgery and home program for 17 mos.; 9 nonretarded children had no surgery over 11-mo. intervening period between testing while 2 had surgery with 22-mo. intervening period between testing	Quick Screening Scale of Mental Development (Motor section)	Progress for retarded children without surgery was 4 mos. less than that for children having surgery, with the latter group having received a longer period of intervention; indicated that the longer the rehabilitation time (between tests), the greater the progress in motor development, particularly for children with no surgery

Study	Sample characteristics	Intensity of intervention program	Instrumentation	Response to treatment and intensity impact
Abdel-Salam, Maraghi, Tawfik[42]	14 children, ages 5 yrs. ± 3 mos.; spasticity (7), postencephalitic, spastic paralysis (7)	1.5 hrs. per session, 6 times weekly for 4 mos.	Clinic-specific assessment	Greater degree of improvement in function, activities of daily living, and perceptual motor performance noted in cp group; noted that treatment provided over time is critical for gains to be realized
Kanda, Yuge, Yamori, Suzuki, Fukase[39]	194 "motor risk" infants <9 mos. of age who had been treated for more than 6 mos.; of 56 children in this group who developed cerebral palsy, 8 children with spastic diplegia treated prior to 9 mos. of age were compared to 21 children with spastic diplegia treated between 9 and 36 mos.	Early treatment group received physiotherapy using Vojta method for mean of 39.3 mos., while late group received training mean of 35.1 mos.	Vojta assessment; CT scans	Treatment effects more pronounced in early treated group with children walking 8 mos. earlier than those in late group
Palmer, Shapiro, Wachtel, et al[2]	48 children, 12–19 mos. of age with mild to severe spastic diplegia	Treatment group received individual 1-hr. sessions every 2 wks. for 12 mos.; contrast groups received 6 mos. of developmental stimulation provided by parents in a home program followed by 6 mos. of therapy.	Bayley scales; standardized neurologic examination	After 6 mos., children receiving therapy only had lower mean motor and mental status than infants in contrast group; differences persisted after 12 mos.; for children with mild to severe spastic diplegia, it was suggested that therapy may not be as effective as home stimulation

Study	Sample characteristics	Intensity of intervention program	Instrumentation	Response to treatment and intensity impact
Wright, Nicholson[12]	47 children, 0–6 yrs. of age; 20 with quadriplegia, 11 with diplegia, and 16 with hemiplegia (5 left and 11 right)	One group acting as controls for 6 mos. followed by 6 mos. therapy; treatment group received 12 mos. of therapy; control group received no treatment	Physical therapy based on the work of Holt (1967) which included function, range of movement, and presence/ absence of primary automatic reflexes; physical and neurologic assessments	Significant differences found in only one subgroup; 7 quadriplegic children receiving therapy progressed signifi- cantly more than their 13 control group counterparts; suggested the importance of therapy for general well-being, social advancement, and happiness of child and family; some children making the least motor progress were more socially aware after therapy than without it
Sommerfeld, Fraser, Hensinger, Beresford[17]	29 severely mentally impaired children, 3–22 yrs. of age; spastic quadriplegia (15), other spastic types (11), athetosis (2), ataxia (1): of this group, 19 children were paired and assigned to either a direct treatment or supervised management group; 10 children acted as control group	Direct treatment group received 2 weekly 30-min. sessions for 5 mos.; supervised manage- ment group received teacher and aide-administered programs	Wilson Developmen- tal Reflex Test; Gross Motor Evaluation	No significant difference found in the development of gross motor skills or increase of passive joint motion among similar studies placed in direct treatment, supervised treatment, or control groups; suggested that less involvement of therapist may be as effective as supervised therapy provided by others

Study	Sample characteristics	Intensity of intervention program	Instrumentation	Response to treatment and intensity impact
Parette[41]	25 children, ages 0–24 mos.; 10 children in experimental group, 2 with spasticity, 1 with athetosis, and 12 with motor delay; 15 children in control group with severe motor delay	Treatment group received individualized levels of treatment for 6 mos.; control group received no therapy	Bayley Scales; Motor Development Evaluation Form	Motor progress of treated groups did not differ significantly from those of control group; in the treated group, motor progress was positively correlated with hours of parental participation and degree of involvement; suggested that therapeutic intervention may obscure the attainment of motor milestones.

CA = chronological age; MA = mental age; MR = mental retardation

Teaming for the future: Integrating transition planning with early intervention services for young children with special needs and their families

Jennifer L. Kilgo, EdD
Coordinator, Graduate Program in
  Early Childhood Special Education
Virginia Commonwealth University
Richmond, Virginia

Nancy Richard, PhD, CCC-SP
Director, Preschool Preparation and
  Transition Project
Hawaii University Affiliated Program

Mary Jo Noonan, PhD
Chairperson
Department of Special Education
University of Hawaii at Manoa
Honolulu, Hawaii

FOR A NUMBER of years the major concern of professionals and advocates was to obtain services for young children who are handicapped or at-risk for handicapping conditions. The passage and implementation of Public Law 99-457 constituted a significant achievement that has resulted in increased emphasis on the continuity of services for young children and their families. The transition or movement of a child from one program or service to the next is a critical event that can be difficult for the child as well as the family. Public Law 99-457 requires that the Individualized Family Service Plan (IFSP) include steps to support the transition of handicapped toddlers to services provided for preschoolers to the extent that such services are considered appropriate. Furthermore, Public Law 99-457 stresses that the IFSP must be developed by a multidisciplinary team and the child's parents.[1]

This federal focus on transition has compelled interest across disciplines. Although the topic has not been emphasized in the literature of related service fields, the issues surrounding transition cross disciplinary boundaries and have relevance to all professionals involved in early intervention.

The purpose of this article is to describe a future-oriented approach to establishing transitioning procedures, some or all of which might be incorporated into interdisciplinary professional practice. The roles of all members of the early intervention team (ie, parents and professionals) in early transitioning and the effects

The model described in this article was developed with funds provided under contract #G008630280, a handicapped children's early education program funded by the US Department of Education, Office of Special Education and Rehabilitation Services. The position statements in this article do not reflect policies of the USDE but are solely the responsibility of the authors, who wish to acknowledge the cooperation of the State of Hawaii Department of Health Infant Development Programs under the direction of Ethel Yamane, Chief, Developmental Disabilities Division.

Inf Young Children 1989; 2(2): 37–48

of parents who become active members in early intervention will be examined. The major focus will be on the need to integrate transition planning throughout the early childhood years. It is hoped that the article will assist the reader in better understanding his or her role, regardless of discipline, when participating in transition planning and programming with families of infants and young children who are at-risk and handicapped.

TRANSITION DURING THE EARLY YEARS

The concept of transition was initially introduced and popularized in the special education literature to address the movement of secondary special education students from school to postschool environments.[2] However, transitions also occur in younger populations, and the concept has expanded to include services for young children. Increased interest in the many issues surrounding transition has been shown by professionals across disciplines. Prevalent transition practices in early intervention services are described in the following section.

Programs and services available

In education and other human service disciplines, the system of services for young children who are at-risk and handicapped has been characterized by a lack of interagency coordination.[3] During the early childhood years, at-risk and handicapped young children and their families are likely to move through a number of special services and agencies, such as neonatal intensive care units, follow-up clinics, public and/or private health care services, infant/family intervention programs, private therapies, public or private day care, and public school services (center-based and/or home-based). Transitions are also likely to occur among various kinds of services within the same agency (eg, from home-based to center-based services). Fig 1 provides a graphic display of the minimum number of transitions that are likely to occur during the first few years of life when a child is at risk or handicapped.

Researchers in early childhood transition models have examined the need for interagency coordination for the timely transfer of records and continuity of services for families. While continuity of services is an important component of early transitions, decisions about subsequent placements are more complex and far-reaching than merely transferring records and intervention plans from the sending program to the receiving program. Instead of focusing on discrete events, transition must be viewed as an ongoing process that includes preparation, implementation, and follow-up.[4] Johnson et al reported that transitions are likely to be more successful if they are well planned, include many opportunities for discussion,

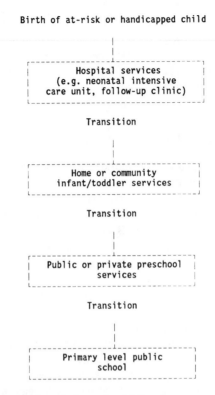

Fig 1. Minimum transitions during early childhood years.

---

involve parents in decision making, and include transition preparation for both young children and their families.[5]

The two most common transitions during early childhood are the transition from infant to preschool programs and the transition from preschool to kindergarten or elementary programs.[6] However, the major work in this area has been directed toward preschool-to-kindergarten transitions. Little emphasis has been placed on transitions from the hospital to the infant program or from the infant program to the preschool program. Beginning in 1986 the Administration for Children, Youth and Families funded 30 projects that addressed early childhood transition practices. A recent listing of handicapped children's early education programs showed 18 funded projects that focused primarily on the transition from preschool to kindergarten; only four projects targeted transitions for the infant population.[7]

Family issues

Although transition issues are faced by families with handicapped children from infancy through adulthood, transition practices have been directed toward the child, with little attention devoted to the family. The question that now confronts professionals across disciplines concerns how early intervention personnel will shift from a more traditional, child-focused model to a family-focused model that includes transition planning as an integrated part of service delivery.

This challenge to let go of established procedures in order to support family members as primary decision makers may be unsettling to early interventionists. Family-focused transition activities (eg, assessment, focused interviewing, collaborative goal setting) require new roles, new skills, and new ways of interacting that extend beyond the expertise of a single discipline. For intervention teams that have already achieved an interdisciplinary or transdisciplinary model, the shift to becoming responsive to and supportive of family strengths and needs during periods of transition should be less difficult. For the large number of early intervention services experiencing personnel shortages,[5] the task of assuming a new set of responsibilities in order to implement transition planning with families may be far more taxing.

THE NEED TO DEVELOP ASSESSMENT, PLANNING, AND IMPLEMENTATION PRACTICES

Public Law 99-457 created new pressures for change in traditional approaches to transition. No systematic procedures have been established to ensure a future-oriented approach to transitions throughout the early childhood years. The legislation reinforces the need to develop a clear definition of transition and to establish assessment, planning, and implementation practices. As interventionists strive to do so, problems and critical professional issues arise that are associated with the process and must be addressed across disciplines:

- How do we define transition?
- Who is to be involved in transition planning?
- Who is responsible for implementation?
- When does transition begin and end?
- How do we determine parent readiness for transition?
- How do we determine the level of parental support?
- How do we implement?
- How do we measure effectiveness?

Interventionists should be aware of these issues and recognize that transition can be a meaningful process that occurs throughout the early childhood years, not simply an event that occurs just before a child leaves a program. Transition must be viewed as a mechanism that prepares both children and families for the next setting.

Readiness for transition

Traditionally, early interventionists have assumed that parents of infants and toddlers with special needs are not ready to begin thinking about the future because of the multitude of immediate concerns regarding their child's medical or developmental status. While certain natural periods of readiness may occur, the assumption that parents of infants and toddlers with special needs are different from the general population in terms of their readiness to consider preschool for their children may not be accurate. Rather than assuming that a parent is ready or not ready, it may be more effective to ask parents to describe their strengths, concerns, and needs for support during the transition process.

Measurement of family strengths and needs

Family assessment models are based on the assumption that parents have differing needs at different times and that effective intervention is tailored to meet individual needs. Recently attention has been focused on the initial assessment of families as they enter early intervention services.[9]

In addition to a more general assessment as families begin to make use of services for their infants, a more specific assessment may be needed to determine the degree of support that parents require for the transition process. Turnbull and Turnbull[10] and, more recently, Dunst et al[11] have discussed the notion of noncontingent help, suggesting that the long-term effects of providing assistance and information that is not requested may foster dependency rather than growth among family members. Professionals must let families know, however, that they are available if assistance is needed. If professionals are to provide the type of assistance that allows families to develop greater skills, particularly in the area of coordination of services for their young children with special needs, assessment is a necessary starting point.

Turnbull[12] has stated that family assessments should be designed to identify and build on family strengths rather than merely to identify needs. If the goal of transition support is to enable parents to become coordinators for their own children, transition assessments should begin with what families are able to do, so that the degree of professional intervention can be adjusted to support families in accomplishing their own goals during the transition process. The purpose of a transition-focused needs assessment, then, is to identify parents' abilities and preferred styles for future planning. The information that both the parents and professionals gain from such an assessment can provide the basis for developing a plan for the future that is individualized for each family.

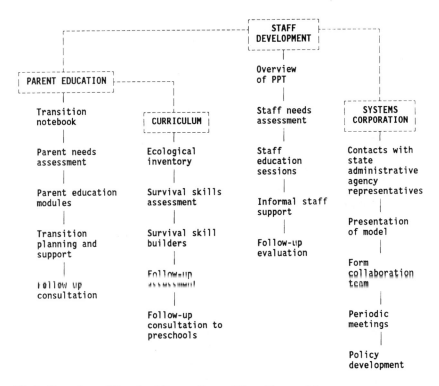

Fig 2. Flow chart of Preschool Preparation and Transition model.

The remainder of this article will present a future-oriented transition model designed to support families of infants and toddlers with special needs in coordinating their transition to preschool. The Preschool Preparation and Transition (PPT) project, a handicapped children's early education program at the University of Hawaii, has been developed and implemented over the past three years in the state of Hawaii. Fig 2 illustrates the four major components of the PPT model: parent education, preparatory curriculum, staff development, and systems cooperation.

PRESCHOOL PREPARATION AND TRANSITION MODEL

One of the major components of the PPT model is parent education, which begins with administration of the Parent Needs Assessment (PNA).[13] The PNA was developed to determine parental preferences, abilities, and need for support during the transition to preschool. The PNA is divided into six topical areas: (1) future planning, (2) need for assistance, (3) need for information, (4) need for support, (5) transition issues, and (6) parental awareness/knowledge. Items in the assessment tool were based on empirical evidence gathered through interview data with professionals and parents in sending and receiving programs, and through literature regarding parents' concerns during early transitions. The areas of greatest concern to parents that emerge from the literature include anxiety about the child's readiness for the next setting, about deciding which type of setting is best, about finding appropriate services for the child in the next setting, and about forming a positive relationship with the receiving teacher.[4,5,14,15] These areas were further validated at the local level in the state of Hawaii to establish the content validity of the PNA. Additional items were designed to assess parents' knowledge of legal rights for children with special needs and of the least-restrictive-environment requirement of Public Laws 94-142 and 99-457.

Measuring family readiness for transition

Development of an assessment tool does not address the questions of when transition-focused assessment should occur and who is competent to administer an interview related to future planning. These questions have surfaced repeatedly at the demonstration sites for the PPT model. The first question (ie, when to approach parents regarding future planning) was addressed systematically.

Data collected in Hawaii between January 1987 and June 1988 from 77 mothers and 31 fathers were analyzed using chi-squares to find patterns in the times when parents were ready to begin planning for preschool. Positive parental responses to questions such as "Have you thought about preschool for your child?" were considered to be evidence of readiness to begin planning for preschool. Significant patterns were observed in mothers' responses, but not in those of fathers. A significantly greater number of mothers responded "yes" when asked about planning for preschool when their children were between the ages of 24 and 29 months. No such pattern emerged for fathers, whose positive responses were evenly spread over age ranges for the children (from 0 to 36 months and older). Fig 3 illustrates the significant increase in mothers' positive responses when their children were between 24 and 35 months of age.

Age of the child was not the only predictor of parents' readiness to consider preschool, however. Further analysis was conducted to determine the relationship between the severity of the child's special needs and parents' readiness to consider preschool.

A rating system was used by which two professionals within the infant program were asked to rate each child's condition thus: 1—at risk/normal, 2—mild, or 3—severe. Reliability was established at an average of 93% agreement between the two observers. Significant patterns were found (via chi-square analysis) for both

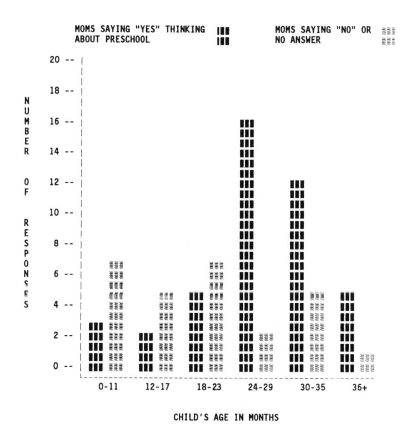

Fig 3. Mothers' readiness to plan for preschool related to the age of the child.

mothers and fathers to indicate an inverse relationship between the severity of the child's special needs and parental readiness to think about the next educational program. Parents of children who were assigned a rating of "3" (severe) by professionals in the infant program responded negatively to questions about preschool planning significantly more often than did parents of children who were rated "1" (at risk/normal) or "2" (mild). Table 1 shows the relationships between ratings of the child's degree of special needs and parental readiness to plan for preschool.

What are the implications of these data for professionals who want to assist families to prepare gradually for the transition to preschool? Foremost is the need to become sensitive to parents' cues, questions, and responses to questions about the future. While a clear "readiness period" was found for mothers around the child's second birthday, some parents indicated readiness to plan earlier while

Table 1. Parents' readiness to consider preschool related to severity of children's needs

Infants' severity rating	Mothers' responses (n = 77)			Fathers' responses (n = 31)		
	N.A.	No	Yes	N.A.	No	Yes
At risk/normal	2	5	18*	1	0	7**
Mild	5	8	24*	4	5	7**
Severe	0	9	6	0	5	2

* = 10.26, df = 4 (p < 0.25)
** = 10.79, df = 4 (p < .025)

others were not ready even as the third birthday approached. The severity of the child's needs certainly emerges as an important variable to consider in addition to the child's age. Both of these variables represent general anchoring points that can serve as reminders to professionals when introducing future planning at any level with family members. Beyond these general patterns, however, individual differences in families indicate that professional assumptions about the readiness of given families to address the future may be unfounded.

A second issue regarding the assessment of parents' need for education and support during the transition process is that of professional roles and responsibilities. Traditionally the social worker or another designated person within an early intervention program has been most likely to discuss future educational placements with the family. This separation of roles interposes a boundary between current programming for the child and family and planning for subsequent educational and community environments. Although certain tasks may be best performed via the direct involvement of a social worker, future planning is related to every aspect of services for young children with special needs and their families. Professionals and paraprofessionals of all disciplines can develop sensitivity to parents' signals and integrate future planning with the services they provide to young children. The PNA is designed to be conducted by any member of the team.

Building on parents' strengths

Particular skills that parents should possess in order to deal with transitions include a thorough knowledge of the child's needs and an ability to state these needs to professionals in sending and receiving agencies. Awareness of the options available in the community is also important so that parents or other key family members can make decisions about the most appropriate options for early educational placement. Noonan and Kilgo[4] described critical skills that parents need to coordinate services for their children, including knowledge of the legal rights of children with special needs and familiarity with a preparatory curriculum and the IFSP process.

Every contact between parents and intervention staff is an opportunity to support parents as the key decision makers for their children. Professionals can acquire transition support skills and integrate these skills into all levels of assessment, programming, and intervention with families.

Transition support skills are actually a specific application of family-focused intervention and as such are consistent with the principles presented most recently by Dunst et al.[11] Specific transition skills include effective communication with family members; knowledge of community resources, of referral timelines for receiving programs, and of skills required in subsequent environments for children; and the ability to work on a team with parents and other staff members.[7] The box provides examples of transition skills often needed by parents and professionals.

Through systematic assessment, professionals can become more sensitive to the transition skills that parents already possess. The context of an early intervention program provides repeated opportunities for parents to acquire transition skills. During the time when parents attend an infant program, professionals can enable parents to function as team members and to take an active role in assessment and programming for their infants. Preparation for transition can be embedded within the intervention process and can be made explicit as soon as parents give an indication of readiness to begin preparing for the next environment beyond the infant intervention program.

Supporting independence

Subsequent to identifying parents' strengths for transition planning, professionals can support parents so as to increase their degree of independence gradually. Each member of the intervention team can interact with family members in a way that is consistent with the principle of enabling parents to become coordinators for their own children. The degree to which individual families are able to coordinate and to make decisions will vary across families, depending on the resources and

---

Transition Skills Needed by Parents and Professionals

Skills parents need	Skills professionals need
• Thorough knowledge of the child's needs	• Effective communication skills
• Ability to state child's needs	• Knowledge of community resources
• Awareness of placement options	• Awareness of referral timelines
• Knowledge of legal rights	• Knowledge of a preparatory curriculum
• Knowledge of a preparatory curriculum	• Knowledge of skills required in subsequent environment
• Knowledge of the IEP/IFSP process	• Teaming skills

skills of each family member. The assumption that each family is able to participate will necessarily permeate all professional interactions with families. An example of preparing for transition as part of early intervention follows:

> Anna attended the early intervention program weekly with her 2-year-
> old daughter, Carrie, who was diagnosed as having general develop-
> mental delays related to seizure activity during the first 6 months of her
> life. Anna's greatest concern with respect to Carrie's development had
> to do with her puzzling habit of tilting her head to look at the world.
> Both the occupational therapist and physical therapist worked exten-
> sively to provide Anna with activities to encourage neck righting. Frus-
> trated after several months and little change in Carrie's habitual head
> tilt, Anna discussed her concerns with the therapy staff at the early inter-
> vention program. Both therapists supported Anna in seeking the opinion
> of an ophthalmologist. Anna expressed her preference for contacting the
> physician on her own and was furnished with copies of her daughter's
> current progress reports in order to expedite the process. She initiated
> and coordinated the referral on her own, discussing the process with the
> therapists at the early intervention program each week. Anna success-
> fully obtained consultation from the ophthalmologist and surgery was
> recommended.

While this example may seem minor, the underlying principle of enabling is
crucial to the development of transition skills. Anna was able to coordinate further
services for her child, and the professionals involved were sensitive to the importance of following her lead and supporting her initiative.

The role of parents on the intervention team

Parent involvement in the assessment process can begin with the initial contact
with the family. Administering the Ecological Inventory provides one means of
beginning to work with parents as partners in assessment. The Ecological Inventory format that is used as part of the PPT model was adapted and shortened for
use with parents and key family members of infants with special needs. The parental interview format requires that the professional assist the parent in describing
each step of daily routines that involve the child (eg, bathing, feeding, dressing,
playtime, nap, bedtime). Both home and community environments are included in
the inventory, providing the opportunity for parents to examine the child's degree
of participation in daily activities. The resulting information can provide the basis
for developing functional goals and objectives that fit into natural contexts for the
child.

The need for every team member to be aware of a functional focus and to incorporate contextual skills into all of their interventions with young children requires

coordinated planning and intervention across the team. Parents are the most consistently involved members of the team. In order to support parents in this role, professionals may spend part of each intervention session devoted to revising plans and soliciting direction from the parents to determine the approach that will best fit into the family routine. Regardless of which team members are present, time can be devoted to providing information about intervention plans in relation to the changing strengths, needs, and preferences of individual families.

Parent education

More formal parent education regarding the transition process can occur when parents express an interest. The PPT model offers five modules that can be sequenced according to parental preference. Topics addressed include

- What's in a transition?
- Legal rights for children with special needs
- Preparing my child for independence
- Who is the transition coordinator?
- Parents and the individualized education program (IEP) meeting

Implementation of parent education at PPT demonstration sites between 1987 and 1988 was conducted primarily via individual sessions, with some small groups, and was supplemented by summary booklets. Parents at two of the demonstration sites completed differing numbers of modules according to individual preference and need for information.

FUTURE PLANNING AND THE IFSP

One component of the proposed IFSP is the transition plan. Although the word "transition" is used somewhat narrowly to mean movement between intervention programs for handicapped children, future-focused planning should be incorporated into both child-related and family-related goals at all levels of early intervention. For example, the results of the Parent Needs Assessment may indicate that parents of a child with a severe handicap wish to meet with other parents who have similar concerns about their children. A future-focused goal for this couple could be simply that they will telephone another family who has indicated a willingness to meet with them. As for the child, he or she may show a willingness to interact socially but may become very aggressive toward other children when made to take turns at given activities. A future-focused goal could then be developed by the parents to increase gradually the time that the child is required to wait for given activities.

Transition planning, while only one component of the IFSP, can provide a focal point for the family and professionals so that every goal and objective contained within the IFSP can address future as well as immediate priorities. The development of independence in home, school, and community environments should be a consideration when writing meaningful goals and objectives.[16] The preparatory focus of the IFSP can be organized around an ongoing transition perspective, instead of viewing transition issues as addenda to the IFSP.

Transition goals in the IFSP

The need for flexibility of family goals has been emphasized repeatedly by several authors in recent discussions of the family-focused intervention.[11,16] Transition planning, as an integral part of the IFSP, must also be flexible and responsive to individual family needs. Table 2 summarizes information gathered via the PNA and resulting goals that were developed jointly by parents and professionals. It is highly likely that changing parental priorities and needs will dictate modification of the initial goals. Periodic review and updating with parents is necessary to maintain an accurate reflection of parental preferences.

Table 2. Parental goals developed from the Parent Needs Assessment

Area addressed on PNA	Parent preference/goal
1. Readiness to plan for preschool	"Not ready. Want to wait another 6 months."
2. Types of preschools considered	"Have not looked at preschools. Want to visit neighborhood preschools with professional support." *Goal: Parent will visit three preschools in last 6 months of infant program.*
3. Assistance in choosing a preschool	"Want phone numbers and an outsider's opinion." *Goal: Parent will call and set up preschool visits; professional to accompany on visits.*
4. Areas in which more information is desired	"Want to discuss shunt with physician and how to notice signs of dysfunction." *Goal: Parent will prepare questions ahead of time with infant program staff and then visit physician.*
5. Need for contact with other parents	"Not interested at this time."
6. Preference for preschool planning approach	"Prefer individual information and planning sessions."
7. Topics of interest	"Want to learn what skills my child will need in preschool." *Goal: Parent will complete module #3, "Preparing My Child for Independence."*

Validation of the PPT model

The model proposed here is currently being field tested, with evaluation in progress. Many questions remain regarding how much of the coordination of transitions parents should be expected to perform on their own and when the actual steps toward a transition should begin. The individualized approach that we have presented was validated for families who participated in the demonstration project in Hawaii between 1986 and 1988. Participants reflected the many ethnic groups in Hawaii, including caucasian, black, Chinese, Filipino, Japanese, Korean, part-Hawaiian, Portuguese, Vietnamese, and Pacific Islanders. Replication activities with the PPT model began in the Richmond, Virginia, area in 1988. Families and professionals in two infant programs there will participate in evaluation and adaptation of the processes and tools developed in Hawaii. To date, evaluation data collected from parents support the integration of future-focused intervention with traditional child-focused services as a means toward a family-focused approach. Four key features of a future-focused model at the infant/toddler program level are (1) transition as a continuous process; (2) teamwork among parents and professionals from all disciplines; (3) individualized support for families; and (4) programming of functional skills for young children.

•   •   •

Traditionally transition to the next program could be mentioned at any time from 6 months to 1 year prior to a family's departure from an infant program. As the authors have advocated, this approach may contribute to the fragmentation of services for families, because transition is viewed as a discrete event rather than as an ongoing process. Through early introduction of future planning, movement to the next environment can be approached gradually and with sufficient preparation of children and their parents.

Teaming with parents is also a gradual process, one that begins with the first contact with a family. Approaching parents and primary caregivers as the key decision makers regarding intervention services and educational programming for their young special-needs children is an initial step toward placing parents in the central role on the intervention team. Family assessment and the development of the IFSP provide the context for a future-focused plan, one that integrates both functional goals for infants/toddlers and transition goals for parents. Each team member who is involved in the implementation of the IFSP has multiple opportunities to encourage parents to coordinate services for their infants independently. Professional sensitivity to individual parents' abilities and preferences in regard to implementing and changing their own goals is needed across disciplines.

In order to provide individualized support, specific transition skills can be acquired by every professional who interacts with parents. These skills include an understanding of family-focused intervention and the steps in transition planning; supporting independence in parents and children; accessing information for parent education; knowledge of community resources; and consultation with receiving educational and community programs.

Functional goals for infants/toddlers are, by definition, preparation to participate more independently in present and future environments. Parental involvement is particularly important to assess the child's degree of participation in present environments and routines at home and in the community. The priorities and needs of each family affect the child's degree of participation. An Ecological Inventory offers one means to support parents in assessing their own children in the context of daily routines and thereby increasing their own observational skills. More formal assessment data can then be integrated with a view toward supporting parents' preferred ways for their children to become more independent in daily routines, thus linking assessment and programming to functional goals and objectives.

As family assessment models and procedures for developing and implementing the IFSP emerge, a future-focused orientation is proposed. Instead of seeking to identify a time when families are ready to begin planning for transition, future planning can be integrated into all levels of interaction with families and their young children with special needs. The processes and tools developed through model demonstration projects such as the PPT model offer a means of addressing parents' concerns for the future in a manner that is responsive to individual differences in strengths, needs, and readiness for planning.

REFERENCES

1. *Education of the Handicapped Act Amendments of 1986.* (22 Sept 1986). *Congressional Record* 132(125), H7893–7912.

2. Ianacone RN, Stodden RA, eds: *Transition Issues and Directions.* Reston, Va, Council for Exceptional Children, 1987.

3. Hutinger P: Transition practices for handicapped young children: What the experts say. *J Div Early Child* 1981;2:8–14.

4. Noonan MJ, Kilgo JL: Transition services for early age individuals with severe mental retardation, in Ianacone RN, Stodden RA, eds: *Transition Issues and Directions.* Reston, Va, Council for Exceptional Children, 1987, pp 25–37.

5. Johnson TE, Chandler LK, Kerns GM, et al: What are parents saying about family involvement in school transitions? A retrospective transition interview. *J Div Early Child* 1986;11:10–17.

6. Bailey DB: Assessing critical events, in Bailey DB, Simeonsson RJ, eds: *Family Assessment in Early Intervention.* Columbus, Ohio, Charles E Merrill, 1988.

7. Administration for Children, Youth and Families: *Transition: Preschool to Kindergarten.* Washington, DC, US Department of Health and Human Services, 1988.

8. Meisels SJ, Harbin G, Modagliani K, et al: Formulating optimal state early childhood intervention policies. *Except Child*, to be published.

9. Bailey DB, Simeonsson RJ, Winton PJ, et al: Family focused intervention: A functional model for planning, implementing, and evaluating individualized family services in early intervention. *J Div Early Child* 1986;10:156–171.

10. Turnbull AP, Turnbull RH: *Parents Speak Out: Then and Now*. Columbus, Ohio, Charles E Merrill, 1985.

11. Dunst CJ, Trivette CM, Deal AG: *Enabling and Empowering Families*. Cambridge, Mass, Brookline Press, 1988.

12. Turnbull AP: Accepting the challenge of providing comprehensive support to families. Read before the International Conference on Mental Retardation, sponsored by the Council for Exceptional Children, Honolulu, Hawaii, Jan 11–13,1988.

13. Noonan MJ, Stodden RA: The preschool preparation and transition model: Preparing handicapped infants for least restrictive environments (technical proposal, US Office of Special Education project No. 024RH60073). Honolulu, Hawaii, University of Hawaii Department of Special Education, 1986.

14. Fowler S: Transition from preschool to kindergarten for children with special needs, in Allen KE, Goet EM, eds: *Early Childhood Education: Special Problems, Special Solutions*. Rockville, Md, Aspen Publishers, 1982, pp 309–330.

15. Gallaher J, Maddox M, Edgar E: *Early Childhood Interagency Transition Model*. Seattle, Wash, University of Washington Experimental Education Unit, 1984.

16. Bailey DB: Considerations in developing family goals, in Bailey DB, Simeonsson RJ, eds: *Family Assessment in Early Intervention*. Columbus, Ohio, Charles E Merrill, 1988, pp 229–250.

The challenge of providing quality group child care for infants and young children with special needs

Marcia Hartley, MS
Research Associate

Claire White, MS

Michael W. Yogman, MD
Assistant Professor
Department of Pediatrics
Harvard Medical School
Boston, Massachusetts

WORKING PARENTS of infants and young children with physical, cognitive, or emotional disabilities, or who are at high biologic or social risk, have a particular need to find high quality, affordable child care for their children. Most mothers of young healthy children work because of economic necessity.[1] Parents of disabled children often need to be employed because of the increased financial burden. The reasons for this financial burden are well known; the medical care, special equipment, and added transportation costs for a variety of appointments often exceed most insurance coverage. The extra pressure on time and economic resources to the family with a disabled child could be ameliorated if quality, affordable child care was more readily available to them. Moreover, young children who are disabled benefit from peer group experiences in the same ways that nondisabled children do.[2]

The 10th Annual Report to Congress on the Education of the Handicapped Act in 1986 recorded the number of handicapped children ages 0 to 21 years in the United States as 4,421,601. Of this total 332,915 were ages 3 to 5.[3] Although data have never been collected on the 0-to-3 age group, one could extrapolate from the 3-to-5-year data and estimate that 450,000 children ages 0 to 3 were handicapped in the United States. Fewell estimated that there were over 2 million handicapped children under age 6.[4]

According to the 10th Annual Report to Congress 265,447 children ages 3 to 5 were being served in special education programs, 8,041 of them in Massachusetts. The remaining 67,468 disabled 3 to 5 year-olds were unserved in any program.[3] In 1985 to 1986, 32,693 children ages 0 to 2 in all 50 states were being served in special education programs. Massachusetts served 2,881 of these children.[5] By fiscal year 1988 the Massachusetts Department of Public Health, which administers early intervention programs in Massachusetts, reported serving 7,000 children ages 0 to 3 with special needs, 35% of whom were deemed to be at environmental risk. Another 1,000 children known to be in need of services remained on waiting lists. According to the Department of Public Health in a telephone conversation in January 1988, approximately 24,000 children ages 0 to 3 years in Massachusetts are in need of services in 1989. Despite increasing national concern for the well-being of disabled children ages 0 to 3, statistical tables rarely differentiate this age group, often overlapping age groups (ie, 0 to 3 years, 2 to 5 years, and 0 to 5 years),

Inf Young Children 1989; 2(2): 1–10

making it difficult to compare statistics. No nationwide system reports the incidence of physical disabilities and mental retardation in this age group, nor do uniform reporting criteria exist even for disabilities and risk conditions that can be identified in the newborn.[6]

Statistics are not available for the number of families of disabled children with two employed parents; however, extrapolating from Fewell's[4] research, and assuming that statistics on maternal employment for the general population apply, a conservative estimate of over 600,000 families with disabled children ages birth to 3 would need child care in order that the parents could work and meet their financial needs. (In 1986 54% of women with children under the age of 6 were working [an increase of approximately 10% each decade since 1948]. The number of employed married women with infants had risen from 31% in 1975 to 50% in 1985. Sixty-four percent of black mothers with infants [under age 1] were employed, which was 15 percentage points higher than the rate for white mothers. Single-parent mothers were more likely to be employed and to work full-time than married mothers, since they provided the full support of their families.[7])

Very little data exist on the availability of child care for infants and toddlers, particularly in family day care homes, and less is known about the availability of child care for disabled children. The Children's Defense Fund cites a "dearth of affordable child care" for all children, which forces parents to compromise on quality and to use a patchwork of child care arrangements.[8] Parents of disabled children report an even more critical lack of availability of organized day care for their children. Of a total day care enrollment of 94,919 in 1988 in Massachusetts, only 2,211 special needs slots existed in the 1,909 licensed centers in Massachusetts to serve all children birth to age 5.[9] This number of special needs slots does not necessarily reflect the number of children with special needs enrolled at a given time, since some slots may not be filled. Of the total enrollment of 94,919 in day care in Massachusetts, 1,559 were infant slots, 6,515 were toddler slots, and 86,845 were preschool slots. With only 2,211 slots for infants, toddlers, and preschool-age children with special needs in Massachusetts, parents not fortunate enough to find high quality family day care or helpful relatives must choose between not working and inadequate child care. More data are needed on the cost and quality of child care services used by special needs children, and on the parents' financial burden and employment status.

The Education of the Handicapped Act Amendments of 1986 (Public Law 99-457) will gather data on the needs of children, ages birth to 3, who are delayed in one or more of the following areas: "cognitive development, physical development, language and speech development, psychosocial development, self-help skills, or who have a diagnosed physical or mental condition which has a high probability of resulting in developmental delay."[10(p1146)] Under Public Law 99-457 each state is encouraged to "develop and implement a statewide, comprehensive, coordinated, multidisciplinary, interagency program of early intervention services for handicapped infants and toddlers and their families."[10(p1147)] Federal funding, however, totaled only $50 million nationally for fiscal year 1987–1988. Most of these early intervention programs do not include child care for the remaining hours of the week that the child is not attending the early intervention program. According to the Department of Public Health, six early intervention programs in Massachusetts have an association with day care centers that provide an extended day program for children with special needs. The Massachusetts Department of Public Health has not surveyed to determine the number of children receiving early intervention services in Massachusetts who are in need of additional child care, but recognizes the need to do so.

TYPES OF EARLY CHILDHOOD PROGRAMS

The major types of child care available to disabled children are center-based care serving only disabled children (segregated centers), integrated center-based care serving both disabled and nondisabled children (integrated centers), family day care, and individual care by relative or babysitter in the child's home or in the caregiver's home. If the disabled child is also in an early intervention program, the day may be divided between the early intervention center-based program and an additional child care setting: a family day care program, a regular day care center, or at home with a caregiver. In the United States, recent statistics for nondisabled preschoolers suggest that approximately 33% of the children ages 0 to 3 are cared for in their own home, and 42% are cared for out of the home, either by a relative or other caregiver. Only 5% of children under 1 year of age are cared for in day care centers. Eleven and seven tenths percent of children ages 1 to 2, and 21% of children ages 3 to 4 are cared for in center-based programs.[11]

All parents want their children to receive the best possible care. While Belsky[12] has raised questions about the adverse effects of out-of-home care for infants, the data he reviews are from self-selected samples rather than randomized trials. Studies with older children suggest that quality of care rather than the particular setting better predict developmental outcome. Recent data from high quality centers in Sweden refute Belsky's contention that early entry is detrimental. Swedish children entering high quality group care prior to age 1 did better on cognitive and socioemotional outcomes at age 8 than children staying at home or entering group care later.[13]

CHALLENGES: AFFORDABILITY AND QUALITY

Challenges to be met in providing more child care slots for disabled children involve maintaining affordable care for families and fair wages for staff without sacrificing quality for children.

Day care is expensive, because it is labor intensive. Salaries comprise the largest percentage of the day care budget. In order to keep the cost of day care within the reach of parents, low child–adult ratios and fair wages for day care staff are often sacrificed. As a result, the quality of care suffers. When the salaries of day care staff are not competitive with the salaries of other competing professions, there is a rapid staff turnover. The importance of having a high quality, stable staff who are paid at a competitive level with other professions cannot be disputed. The tension between these three highly related day care issues—quality for children, affordability for parents, and fair wages for staff—has been called the "child care trilemma."[14] The solution to the policy trilemma is that child care will need to be subsidized from both public and private sources in order that children not be subjected to substandard care.

QUALITY IN REGULAR GROUP CARE

The need for high quality group care is the same for disabled and for nondisabled children. In order to provide comprehensive, integrated services to children with special needs, particular attention must be given to group size and child–adult ratio, developmentally appropriate activities for the children, specialized staff training and supervision, and protected time for communication with parents. Bredekamp[15] and Godwin and Schrag[16] have provided guidelines for caregiving recommended by the National Association for the Education of Young Children. These guidelines describe developmentally appropriate care of infants, toddlers, and preschoolers in a variety of day care settings.

GROUP SIZE AND RATIOS

A low child–adult ratio and small group size are both critically important for quality infant and toddler day care according to a national day care study, although group size was found to be a more important variable in the quality of care for preschool children.[17] The need of the very young child to have more individualized attention, and the need for the preschool child not to be lost in a large group of children, requires a larger staff than at the elementary school level. Obviously the disabled child may need even more individualized attention. All states have regulations that determine group size and ratio, and some states require special needs licenses to serve special needs children. However, there is tremendous variability from state to state as shown in Table 1.[18]

A state license, therefore, is certainly helpful, but is not a sufficient guarantee of quality. For example, for a child age birth to 18 months, Maryland requires a child–adult ratio of 3:1. Idaho allows a ratio of 12:1, and South Carolina allows a ratio of 8:1. For a child age 18 to 30 months, Maryland requires a child–adult ratio of 6:1, while Idaho and South Carolina allow a ratio of 12:1. At age 30 to 36

Table 1. Day care licensing requirements

| States | Day care centers child-to-staff ratios | | | | | Family day care homes |
	0–12 months	12–18 months	18–24 months	24–30 months	30–36 months	# allowed in home
Alabama	6:1	6:1	6:1	10:1	10:1	6
Alaska	5:1	6:1	6:1	10:1	10:1	6
Arizona	5:1	6:1	6:1	10:1	10:1	4
Arkansas	6:1	6:1	9:1	12:1	12:1	16
California	4:1	4:1	4:1	4:1	12:1	12
Colorado	5:1	5:1	5:1	5:1	8:1	6
Connecticut	4:1	4:1	4:1	4:1	10:1	6
Delaware	4:1	7:1	7:1	10:1	10:1	6
District of Columbia	4:1	4:1	4:1	8:1	8:1	5
Florida	6:1	8:1	12:1	12:1	15:1	5
Georgia	7:1	7:1	10:1	12:1	15:1	6
Hawaii	prohibited	prohibited	prohibited	8:1	16:1	5
Idaho	12:1	12:1	12:1	12:1	12:1	6
Illinois	4:1	5:1	8:1	8:1	10:1	8
Indiana	4:1	5:1	5:1	7:1	10:1	10
Iowa	4:1	4:1	4:1	6:1	8:1	6
Kansas	3:1	5:1	7:1	7:1	12:1	10
Kentucky	6:1	6:1	6:1	10:1	12:1	12
Louisiana	6:1	8:1	12:1	12:1	14:1	*
Maine	4:1	5:1	5:1	8:1	10:1	12
Maryland	3:1	3:1	6:1	6:1	10:1	6
Massachusetts	3:1	4:1	4:1	10:1	10:1	6
Michigan	5:1	9:1	9:1	12:1	12:1	6
Minnesota	4:1	7:1	7:1	7:1	10:1	14
Mississippi	5:1	9:1	12:1	12:1	14:1	15
Missouri	4:1	4:1	8:1	8:1	10:1	10
Montana	4:1	4:1	4:1	8:1	8:1	6
Nebraska	4:1	4:1	6:1	6:1	10:1	8
Nevada	4:1	6:1	6:1	6:1	7:1	6
New Hampshire	4:1	5:1	6:1	6:1	8:1	6
New Jersey	4:1	4:1	7:1	7:1	10:1	5
New Mexico	6:1	6:1	10:1	10:1	12:1	12
New York	4:1	4:1	4:1	4:1	6:1	6
North Carolina	7:1	7:1	7:1	12:1	12:1	5
North Dakota	4:1	4:1	4:1	5:1	5:1	7
Ohio	5:1	6:1	7:1	8:1	12:1	12
Oklahoma	4:1	6:1	6:1	8:1	12:1	5
Oregon	4:1	4:1	4:1	10:1	10:1	5
Pennsylvania	4:1	4:1	5:1	5:1	10:1	6
Rhode Island	4:1	4:1	4:1	4:1	4:1	6

continues

Table 1. continued

	Day care centers child-to-staff ratios					Family day care homes
States	0–12 months	12–18 months	18–24 months	24–30 months	30–36 months	# allowed in home
South Carolina	8:1	8:1	12:1	12:1	15:1	6
South Dakota	5:1	5:1	5:1	5:1	10:1	12
Tennessee	5:1	7:1	8:1	8:1	10:1	7
Texas	5:1	6:1	9:1	11:1	15:1	12
Utah	4:1	4:1	7:1	7:1	15:1	6
Vermont	4:1	4:1	4:1	5:1	5:1	6
Virginia	4:1	5:1	5:1	10:1	10:1	9
Washington	4:1	7:1	7:1	10:1	10:1	6
West Virginia	4:1	4:1	4:1	8:1	8:1	7
Wisconsin	4:1	4:1	4:1	6:1	8:1	8
Wyoming	5:1	5:1	8:1	8:1	10:1	6

Reprinted with permission from Binder A, Chapiro B. Licensed to care. *Parenting* 1988;2(7):72–74.
© 1988 Parenting Magazine.

months, there is again a great disparity in the standards from state-to-state. Low child–staff ratios are especially important for infants and toddlers, allowing caregivers to spend less time simply managing children and taking care of basic needs. The Abt study also reported that infants and toddlers cry less in groups in which there are fewer children, and are more talkative, innovative, and involved in their play.[17]

A POSITIVE EARLY CHILDHOOD ENVIRONMENT

Caregivers in early childhood programs, both center-based and family-based, typically stress social development: sharing, waiting to take a turn, learning to play with others, understanding the feelings and respecting the rights of others, learning to take initiative, learning to ask for help, learning cooperative and non-aggressive ways of interacting with peers, and developing a feeling of well-being and self-worth. Many of the daily activities of infants and toddlers require a variety of skills, which allows children at various developmental levels to participate, including children with special needs. Activities such as play dough, painting, music, as well as sand, water, and block and dramatic play are enjoyed by disabled children as much as they are enjoyed by children of many developmental levels, with or without disabilities. Caregivers who understand early childhood education will emphasize the enjoyment of the experience and not the product of the child's efforts.

In a comparison of environments for preschool children and staff, Bailey, Clifford, and Harmes[19] found that centers with only disabled preschool children (segregated centers) had fewer activities and areas that would foster creativity and social development. Mealtime at child care centers with only nondisabled children were much more likely to be a time for encouraging socialization and self-help skills.[20] A better understanding of the disabled child's strengths would aid the staff in normalizing the environment. Adjustments to the environment that include providing accessible, comfortable space that facilitates social and physical development, as well as independence, are necessary for the disabled child to thrive in integrated group care. Changes to an ordinary day care environment may include increased space to accommodate adaptive equipment for the disabled child, spatial arrangements that encourage independence, and space for social interactions.[5]

STAFF QUALIFICATIONS, TRAINING, AND SUPERVISION

The National Association for the Education of Young Children recommends that early childhood teachers have "college-level specialized preparation in early childhood education/child development,"[21] as well as supervised, practical experience with young children. At the present time, day care regulations in most states require a teacher to have only a high school diploma and limited experience with children. The use of untrained, inexperienced teachers places an extra burden of training and supervision on other day care staff. Ongoing observation, feedback, and support of the staff are necessary in providing supervision. Through regularly scheduled discussions of problems, as well as individual supervision, staff with less experience can be trained.

When serving disabled young children, supervisors need special expertise and access to consultants for special problems. The staff need to be fully informed about the child's special condition and special needs. Also, detailed health and safety policies need to be established, and staff training must be ongoing.

Inservice training should be tailored to the needs of the staff. Sessions should include pertinent topics such as strategies for integrating disabled children in activities, communication with parents and professionals, information about disabilities and how the disability may affect the child's ability to learn or to participate. Staff development programs give the support that individual family child care providers often lack. A special training project in Michigan for family child care providers focused on using physical space for enhancing the child's development, attitudes toward disabled children, and programming for children with special needs.[22] Six months after the start of the training, the trainees' attitudes toward handicapped children, knowledge of programming for the disabled, and utilization of physical space for enhancing growth and development were compared with the pretraining levels. The training included workshops on caring for children with special needs, a resource file on child development and how it is affected by various handicapping conditions, visits to the trainees' family day care homes for consultation and support, consultation by medical and educational professionals, and technical assistance to family day care organizations. Results demonstrated a significant positive change overall for the trainees from pre- to posttraining.[22]

COMMUNICATION WITH PARENTS

No one is as familiar with the child's needs and accomplishments as the parents, and this information from parents should be shared with the members of the educational team before the child enters the program and as frequently as possible thereafter through formal and informal channels. The casual five-minute chat as the child is left at the day care center can be an important opportunity for discussing the child's progress and needs.[23] Anticipating the child's needs will often prevent unhappy times. For example, knowing that the child will be hungry earlier than usual because of an early breakfast, or seeing that the child needs a quiet time with the caregiver, helps the caregiver plan and provide for the child in a sensitive way. When the parents arrive in the afternoon, the teacher should describe the child's day to them through either in-person or written communication. Careful attention to communication can lessen the competitive feelings that are sometimes felt between parent and caregiver. This level of communication does not always occur in child care programs; however, it is especially important with parents of a child who has special needs, particularly when the child cannot speak. Open communication and cooperation between parent and caregiver, and agreement on goals for the child, require planning and effort from all caregivers, including parents, day care staff, therapists, and medical professionals.

SPECIAL CHALLENGES FOR WORKING WITH SPECIAL NEEDS INFANTS AND TODDLERS IN GROUP CHILD CARE

Staffing

Some states require regular day care centers to have at least a part-time special educator on staff if the center has disabled children enrolled. Centers must decide if staff with a special education background should be hired for direct care of disabled children, or if an off-site or on-site consultant is preferable. The decision is based on the needs and strengths of the day care staff as well as the children. Since special educators command a higher salary than regular day care staff, budgetary implications must be considered.

Planning, communication, and coordination of efforts between the family, day care program, early intervention program or special education program, and other services such as physical therapy, medical, and social services are essential.[24] Extra transportation services may be needed for a child during the middle of the day so that he or she can be moved between programs. It is usually less expensive and often preferable to keep the child in a single setting and to transport staff, such as physical, occupational, and speech therapists. Visiting nurses associations, Easter Seals, and local educational agencies often provide physical therapy in the child's home, but are also willing to provide services in the day care center or family day care home. This arrangement often facilitates the implementation of services, since working parents have difficulty keeping appointments during their work hours. Having therapy in a familiar setting, instead of a clinic, is a less threatening experience for the child. The parents should be included in the session whenever possible and should always be given written information on the therapy session if they were unable to be present. Parents and caregivers may offer suggestions to the therapist of ways to elicit the child's cooperation with therapy. In turn, parents and caregivers learn a great deal from the sessions that they can incorporate in the daily care of the child.

Multidisciplinary team decision making

The multidisciplinary team of medical, educational, and social services must learn to work closely with the family and with each other in order to provide quality care. The genuine desire to provide the best possible care for young children can sometimes elicit territorial feelings among staff, and between staff and parents. The very human tendency of the professional staff to believe they know the best solution or intervention often undermines the validity of the parents' knowledge and common sense. The pressure of accountability for a service being arranged for the child often puts a team member in a defensive position. Tension over status (as demonstrated by salary) of the various team members from medicine, nursing, social work, physical therapy, special education, and early childhood education can be an underlying cause of dissension.

At times the parents' feelings of sadness, anger, or guilt will surface because they may feel safe with the day care staff, and also because there are few other outlets for the parents to express their concerns. This added stress on the staff can cause tension and frustration. Each transition and adjustment of the family and the disabled child require enormous emotional resilience on the part of the family and the day care staff who often become deeply involved. The grief process for the family may be similar to parents' reactions to the birth of their disabled infant or to the loss of a previous pregnancy. Particularly difficult times for parents occur on birthdays, anniversaries of the diagnosis, transition from a program, and when their child does not achieve a developmental milestone. The feelings of sadness or of anger and anxiety can cause great stress. It may be helpful to conceptualize this as a normal developmental progression. An initial period of upset, then denial of the reality of the extent of the child's disability, may be followed by a period of sadness, anger, and anxiety. A gradual adaptation, involving a marshalling of coping skills, is followed by a final phase, reorganization.[25] The positive support provided to the family by the multidisciplinary day care team, and the peer support to each other, can provide a basis for growth and understanding. The team approach may be cumbersome, and filled with opportunity for disagreement, but it offers the best possible avenue for drawing on the strengths of a rich and varied background of experience and knowledge of the staff and family. With experience parents, day care staff, medical, and social service staff can develop effective, supportive methods of communication.

An enormous body of literature exists concerning group decision making. Adhering to these suggestions can facilitate teamwork in many instances. Project Bridge[26,27] provides an excellent method for team members to build skills in decision making. In order to define the problem all members must be fully aware of the child's disability and strengths. Further information gathering that concerns economic and cultural factors, as well as family expectations, must also be considered. Generating alternatives and options for service is a team process of listing possible solutions, with insistence on full team participation. An emphasis on what the child needs, as opposed to the services available, should be of paramount importance. The team must choose one or several of the alternatives as it takes into consideration how each alternative would affect the family and the goals of quality care. A very important part of this step in the decision-making process is to keep accurate records concerning the assignment of responsibilities, the timetable, and procedures for monitoring progress. The subsequent steps of implementing the services, and finally evaluating the services as a team, should lead to a joint determination of success, or the beginning of another process of group information gathering and generating of alternative solutions.

INDIVIDUALIZED CARE FOR THE CHILD AND FAMILY

Decisions about services should be made according to the child's ability to function in the environment, not according to his or her diagnosis. There is tremendous variability even among disabled children with the same diagnosis since an impairment can range from mild to severe. Medical care and community support services that may or may not have been available to the child and family may greatly influence and improve function once they are offered. The multidisciplinary team, which includes parents, should determine the strengths of the child as well as the resources that will be needed to promote his or her development. Amendments to the Education of the Handicapped Act stipulate that each handicapped child receive a "multidisciplinary assessment and identification of appropriate services, and an Individualized Family Service Plan (IFSP), written by a multidisciplinary team and the parent or guardian. The IFSP will contain the infant's and toddler's present levels of physical, cognitive, language and speech, and psycho-social development, as well as self-help skills and the family's strengths and needs."[10(p1150)] Also included are a case manager "from the profession most immediately relevant to the infant's and toddler's or family's needs who will be responsible for the implementation of the plan and coordination with other agencies, and a transition plan to special services at age 3."[10(p1150)]

INTEGRATED GROUP CHILD CARE AND POSSIBLE LIMITS

If the limitations of the child care setting or the limitations of the staff's ability to meet the child's goals cannot be improved, another child care arrangement should be considered. The needs of the nondisabled children in the group should be considered as well. Including a particular disabled child in the group should not be done to the detriment of the group as a whole. All efforts to integrate a child may not be successful. The challenge to the team is to provide the training and support that will enable the staff and parents to accomplish the integration of the disabled child into the center or to find a satisfactory match between the child and a more appropriate child care program. Some disabled children, as well as nondisabled children, thrive in family day care settings and not in large day care centers. The warm, more family-like environment of the family day care home may indeed be the "least restrictive environment" for many children.

SUPPORT OF PARENTS

Another important area of support is to make the parents of the disabled child feel a welcome part of the family day care home or center and parent group. A parent of a disabled child may feel uncomfortable at a parent meeting, and it is common for parents of nondisabled children who have never had the experience of interacting with families of children with handicaps to feel ill-at-ease. The parents of the nondisabled children can be helped to learn about the disability. Staff and parents should be encouraged to facilitate interactions and relationships between all of the families. A variety of parent groups may be successful. Parents of one group (classroom) of children may enjoy meeting as a small group. Other parents prefer a large meeting with a structured program or a performer. Some parents want their children with them, and others prefer to have a social night without the responsibility of their children. Many day care centers find that a dinner, with child care provided at the center, is the most successful type of parent meeting.

• • •

The family of the disabled child has all of the needs of the family of the nondisabled child, with the added problems that are particular to their child's own development. A high quality family day care home or center-based program can reduce the stress and enrich the family's daily existence. Child care professionals and parents who have worked together to provide a supportive environment that is optimal for both children with and without special needs can attest to the benefit to all who participate.

REFERENCES

1. Select Committee on Children, Youth and Families, U.S. Congress: *Demographic and Social Trends: Implications for Federal Support of Dependent-Care Services for Children and the Elderly*, 98th Cong, 2nd sess, Washington, DC, 1984.

2. Rubenstein J, Howes C: The effects of peers on toddler interaction with mother and toys. *Child Dev* 1975;47:597–605.

3. U.S. Department of Education: *10th Annual Report to Congress on the Education of the Handicapped Act*, 1986, Table BA3, pB5 of Appendix B.

4. Fewell R: Child care and the handicapped child, in Gunzenhauser N, Caldwell B, eds: *Group Care of Young Children: Considerations for Child Care and Health Professions, Public Policy Makers, and Parents*. Somerville, NJ, Johnson & Johnson, 1986.

5. U.S. Department of Education: *10th Annual Report to Congress on the Education of the Handicapped Act*, 1986, Table BD1, pB6 of Appendix B.

6. National Center for Clinical Infant Programs: *Infants Can't Wait*. Washington, DC, 1986.

7. Hayghe H: Rise in mothers' labor force activity includes those with infants. *Monthly Labor Rev* 1986;43–45.

8. *A Children's Defense Budget FY 1989*. Washington, DC: 180.

9. Massachusetts Office for Children: *State Summary Sheet for Group Day Care Centers*. Boston, Mass, 1988.

10. Public Law 99-457: *Education of the Handicapped Act Amendments of 1986*, 1146–1150.

11. O'Connell M, Rogers C: Child care arrangements of working mothers: June 1982. *Current Population Reports*. Series P-23, No. 129. Bureau of the Census, Washington, DC, Nov 1983, p 4.

12. Belsky J: Infant day care: A cause for concern? *Zero to Three*, National Center for Clinical Infant Programs, Washington, DC, 1986;6(5):1–7.

13. Anderson B-E: Effects of public day care—Longitudinal study. *Child Dev*, to be published.

14. Morgan G: Supplemental care for young children, in Yogman M, Brazelton T, eds: In *Support of Families*. Cambridge, Mass, Harvard University Press, 1986.

15. Bredekamp S, ed: *Developmentally Appropriate Practice*. Washington, DC, National Association for the Education of Young Children, 1986.

16. Godwin A, Schrag L, eds: *Setting Up for Infant Care: Guidelines for Centers and Family Day Care Homes*. Washington, DC, National Association for the Education of Young Children, 1988.

17. Ruopp R, Travers J, Glantz F, et al: *Children at the Center, Final Report of the National Day Care Study*. Cambridge, Mass, Abt Associates, 1979.

18. Binder A, Shapiro B: Licensed to care. *Parenting* 1988;2(7):72–73.

19. Bailey D, Clifford R, Harmes F: Comparison of preschool environments for handicapped and nonhandicapped children. *Top Early Child Spec Educ* 1982;2(1):9–20.

20. Bailey D, Harmes F, Clifford R: *Top Early Child Spec Educ* 1983;3(2):19–32.

21. Willis A, Ricciuti H: *A Good Beginning for Babies*. Washington, DC, National Association for the Education of Young Children, 1986.

22. Jones S, Meisels S: Training family day care providers. *Top Early Child Spec Educ* 1987;7(1): 1–12.

23. Yogman M: Child care as a setting for parents' education, in Gunzenhauser N, Caldwell B, eds: *Group Care of Young Children: Considerations for Child Care and Health Professions, Public Policy Makers, and Parents*. Somerville, NJ, Johnson & Johnson, 1986.

24. Klein N: Disabled children need day care, too. *Educ Unlimited* 1981;3(1):50–53.

25. Drotar D, Baskiewicz B, Irvin N, et al: The adaptation of parents to the birth of an infant with congenital malformation: A hypothetical model. *Pediatrics* 1975;56:710–717.

26. Spenser P, Coye R: Project Bridge: A team approach to decision-making for early services. *Inf Young Children* 1988;1(1):82–92.

27. Handley E, Spencer P: *Project Bridge: Decision-Making for Early Services: A Team Approach*. Elk Grove Village, Ill, American Academy of Pediatrics, 1986.

Index